Google LDN!

By

Joseph Wouk

Google LDN !

By

Joseph Wouk

ISBN 978-0-578-00439-6

Forward

It is with great pleasure that I write the forward for Joseph Wouk's superb book "Google LDN !" regarding his positive experience in taking Low Dose Naltrexone.

Mr. Wouk writes with enthusiasm, emotion and belief in how taking low dose naltrexone was instrumental in turning his life around when he was suffering with life threatening health issues.

I have been successfully prescribing low dose naltrexone for over twenty years for patients suffering from immune system related disorders.

I am thrilled that Mr. Wouk has chosen to write about his amazing journey in taking this drug.

I thank him very much for his help in spreading this life saving information.

Bernard Bihari, M.D.

New York City

January 2009

For Dr. Bernard Bihari

Acknowledgements

First and foremost to Diane Fenner, whose phone call after more than 20 years saved my life, and who since then has stood by me and helped me through the most difficult period I've ever had to endure.

To Dr. David Gluck, without whose encouragement I might have never completed this project and without whose website I might never have learned the importance of LDN.

To Jon Shemitz who was there to help me at a time no one else would.

To Julia Schopick who encouraged and helped me with the editing.

Finally, to my parents, Herman and Sarah Wouk who gave me the love I needed when I needed it most.

Introduction

The original title of this book was *PLACBO – A Rationalist Seeks a Miracle Cure*.

I started writing it shortly after being diagnosed with Multiple Sclerosis in November 2007. It was originally meant as a journal of my attempt to try to cure myself by going to Peru and finding a Shaman to do an ayahuasca ceremony for my benefit.

As a rationalist, I knew this was silly. But after being told by the best MS doctors on the west coast that there was nothing more they could do for me, I felt I had to at least *try* the Shaman cure. What did I have to lose, after all?

Part One of the book is my own attempt to justify to myself doing this by ascribing any positive results that might happen to the placebo effect. That way I could protect my view of myself as a rationalist even while doing irrational acts. It was written real time as my mind was crumbling from the effects of subcortical dementia; not uncommon among people suffering from my rare subtype of MS, Progressive Relapsing.

And then, completely unexpectedly, ***all my symptoms disappeared*** right before I was scheduled to go to Peru in July.

It turned out that a drug I had been taking as an afterthought; LDN (Low Dose Naltrexone) was the cause of this amazing recovery. I had been taking no other drug at the time. There was no doubt that it was the LDN that had accomplished this.

I had also not expected anything from the LDN, not having bothered to research it. So there's no possibility of it having resulted from the placebo effect, which was what I had been counting on using the Shamanic approach.

The name of the book was changed to *Google LDN!* for two main reasons.

If I had Googled LDN myself, I would have found out about it and gotten relief *before* the MS had had a chance to destroy my life.

Most importantly, though, anyone who sees the title can get the same benefit as if he had purchased the book.

To the passing potential reader, I implore you to do as the title suggests. What you will find out is the best solution to any immune system related disorder that you or an acquaintance may be suffering from.

LDN helps by causing the body to produce three times the normal amount of endorphins. This fortifies the immune system and restores it to its proper working condition. It does this with no side effects or danger to the patient.

Part Two of the book is about my recovery and why it is that twenty years after it was discovered to help immune system disorders LDN remains unknown and unused by most physicians and patients. It's not a pretty story. As usual, the "root of all evil" lies at the core of the problem.

Naltrexone is approved by the FDA for treatment of recovering addicts. It is now a generic drug.

Not enough money can be made from it to justify laying out the millions required to do the double blind studies necessary to get FDA approval for this far more important usage.

Nevertheless, scientific studies from hospitals and Universities around the world are now being published proving that LDN indeed accomplishes what its proponents claim. It's only a question of time before it somehow gets FDA approval. In the meantime it can be prescribed legally as an "off label" use by any doctor willing to do so.

The Appendix will provide the reader with enough credible information to hopefully convince any doctor to go ahead and give the prescription.

My heart and best wishes go out to all those suffering immune system related disorders as I did.

This book is the best I could do to try to help them.

Prologue

"Happy birthday, old Jofess...."

It was my 92-year-old father, Herman Wouk, on the line. It was actually the day after my 54th birthday, but since my dad is an Orthodox Jew he couldn't call me on my actual birthday which was on Saturday.

"How's the new book coming?" he asked.

"Not bad, actually. I've finished the first six chapters, and I've come up with a subtitle for 'In Search of the Placebo effect', 'A Rationalist Seeks a Miracle Cure', what do you think?"

"I like it. So are you planning on detailing how it was that you arrived at this philosophic position?"

"Not really, Pop. I actually meant to use the word way the way it is ordinarily used today, to mean a 'modern outlook' rather than in its philosophic meaning opposing empiricism."

Of course, it was perfectly understandable that my father would assume I meant the philosophical meaning of the word. The last 10 or 15 years I had been deeply involved in studying both philosophy and science. Not in any professional sense, my academic background was in the humanities at Columbia College. I had gone on to finish Columbia Law School.

But I had had a late in life discovery of these two topics, which I had pretty much glossed over while in school. After all of this time studying

I don't know how many books and lectures, I consider myself to be an advanced dilettante in both fields.

But this book is not meant to be an academic exploration of the relationship of rationalism to the miraculous. This book is a story of how a modern man deals with his life when modernity fails to help him solve a major problem.

The problem I face, is multiple sclerosis; a disease which has no cure, and which Western medicine can only guess at the cause.

I was faced with the choice; wait for the disease to do its worst while Western science struggled to understand and overcome it, or try to find some other unconventional way to cure myself.

The problem is that I really am a skeptic. In order to search for an unconventional cure, I will have to leave my rationality behind at some point. It will be a struggle between what I "know" and what I need to learn in order to cure myself.

This book will be a record of my journey to try to find that "miracle cure." It has only just begun and of this writing, I have absolutely no idea how it will end up.

But I hope to bring the reader along, with truth and humor as my guides.

So come along then, let's push the envelope and see if it's possible to do an end run around the consensus reality that all of us buy into.

Whatever happens to me at the end, this life has been a fun and fascinating "E-Ticket" ride for me. Like all E-ticket rides, this one is not recommended for the faint of heart or closed of minds.

But if you can stand it, it's by far and away the best ride in the park.

April 6, 2008

Part One

PLACEBO

A Rationalist Seeks a Miracle Cure

1. *"Your watch is on too tight."*

I stared at my wife in stunned disbelief. She returned my stare followed by a shrug.

This diagnosis was made by the sweet middle-aged lady doctor at the Santa Cruz medical clinic, urgent care.

"I can't see how that makes much sense; I've been wearing this watch for years. It has a Velcro strap, and I never make it too tight..."

The doctor pointed to a slight pink mark that remained where my watch had once been strapped.

"Can't you see? It's left this mark..."

"Yeah, but I really don't see how that could have made my whole arm go numb..."

"Oh, it most certainly can..." She assured me. "Let's see how it feels tomorrow. If it doesn't get better, come back."

On one level, I knew this diagnosis couldn't be right. After all, the problem had begun over a week ago, when the inside of my thumb began to tingle. Then the tingle started spreading to my other fingers. Day by day it kept getting a little worse until the whole hand became numb followed by the inside part of my arm.

But when it comes to health, the old adage "hope springs eternal," comes into play very heavily. I glanced at my wife again, "Who knows? Maybe she's right. That sure would be great if she was..."

Sadly, the "tight watch" diagnosis didn't even make it through the night. By the time I went to sleep, it was already clear to me that I was getting worse even without wearing a watch.

The next day I went to our chiropractor who adjusted me and tried to help. A day later, I was back in his office. His treatment had done nothing to make me better and after trying a few more things he started to look worried. "I don't think this is something I can help you with. Have you got a good M. D.?"

I told him the story of the tight watch. I didn't have my own doctor, only urgent care. He referred me to a doctor he trusted.

It took another two weeks of doctor's appointments before I finally ended up at the neurologist's office. By now, my arm from the shoulder down was completely numb, and unable to function properly. I didn't seem to have any strength in my left-hand at all. I began to drop things all over the place. When I tried to open a can of Coke while holding the can in my left hand, the can broke free from the pressure of trying to open it. It fell on the floor and squirted all over the place.

The only part of my hand I could now feel were the thumb and forefinger. I couldn't really feel anything from them, but they were very stiff. The effect was sort of like having a disembodied lobster claw hanging in front of my body.

After doing a bunch of physical tests, he sent me to have an MRI. The results showed that my brain and spinal cord both had lesions on them. The neurologist told me it looked like I might have multiple sclerosis.

Six years earlier the same neurologist had treated me for a condition called "optic neuritis." One of my eyes had stopped seeing color and was only seeing sepia. He had ordered an MRI then too, but the pictures had come back clean.

Once again, hope springing eternal had been my undoing. When the neurologist told me that the MRI showed neither a brain tumor nor MS lesions I was naturally very relieved. He told me that sometimes, albeit rarely, optic neuritis could show up on its own. He said it should straighten itself out in a couple weeks. What he didn't tell me was what other symptoms to keep my eyes open for in case it *was* MS.

After having spent the previous night praying I had MS rather than a brain tumor, I was so relieved at this news that I just put the whole episode behind me. I didn't do any real research on MS. When the optic neuritis got better, I just forgot about the whole thing.

Three years later my right hand went numb a bit. I went to the chiropractor whose treatment didn't seem to help much, but the condition cleared itself up in two weeks so I once again forgot about it.

The bottom line was that I had been suffering from MS for at least six years without treating it at all.

After four IV infusions of steroids, and three weeks of steroid pills I got back about 70% of the feeling and use of my left hand. This was four months ago and it hasn't gotten any better since. I've had to come to terms with the fact that it probably never will. But that's not all I've had to come to terms with.

Please bear with me here as I tell you about Multiple Sclerosis. I know it's a bummer, but it's important if you are interested in understanding my motivations in this tale.

Multiple sclerosis is currently not curable with western medicine. The scientists don't really know what causes it. The consensus seems to be that it is an autoimmune disease, though a significant number believe it to be something else.

The three standard treatments each offered to reduce the number of relapses by 20 to 30%. A new more dangerous treatment promised a 60% reduction.

I started doing my research in earnest. It looked like I was really pretty screwed. Because I was diagnosed so late (I was 53), and because I was male, the prognosis was particularly bad. Let's see... according to Wikipedia MS patients die on average only eight years younger than healthy people. Great! At least it's not a quick death sentence. Less great, 50% of MS patients die from the disease. Even worse, 15% of MS sufferers die at their own hand.

So basically, it was only a question of time until I would be crippled. If the last attack had hit my leg rather than my arm I already would've been in a wheelchair.

Around the same time as my optic neuritis I had come down with a very heavy case of depression. I realized I was having mental problems when I stood in my closet for five minutes trying to decide what shirt to put on. The problem was I really didn't care what shirt I wore, I just found it impossible to make up my mind.

I did a search for this symptom online and I turned up depression. Me? Depressed? No way. Back then I thought that most cases of depression were simply the result of weak willed people unable to deal with getting old. In fact, I used to joke that depression was a euphemism for being over 45.

Just to be sure, I took an online depression test and I answered honestly. I scored one level above the lowest, which is considered suicidal.

After six months of talk-talk therapy not only was I still depressed, but I began to suffer from awful panic attacks. Finally I got a prescription for Prozac and Xanax which alleviated the worst of the symptoms.

Now, six years later, it was all beginning to make sense. Depression is listed together with optic neuritis as one of the commonest symptoms of MS. Other things began to make sense as well.

For at least six years I had been having problems holding back my urination. From the time I first noticed that I needed to pee till it became an emergency became shorter and shorter. I thought, "Uh oh... prostate!" I went to the urologist expecting to be told I had an enlarged prostate. Instead, he said to me "You have a young man's prostate..."

"Well, then what is causing this pee-pee problem?" I asked.

"It could be a lot of things. Can you handle it?"

"Sure.. No sweat!" I was so relieved to have once again evaded the silver bullet that I left it at that. So every once in a while I have to pull the car over to relieve myself. So what…

Now I was finding out that this was also a classic symptom of MS.

But worst of all I've found out about the cognitive effects of multiple sclerosis.

I had noticed, as had my family and friends, that I had gotten exceptionally absent-minded over the last few years. This wasn't the usual absentmindedness... forgetting where you left the keys or the like. This was walking into a room to do something and suddenly realizing you had no idea why you were there. The only way I could figure out what it was to re-trace my steps in to the room from which I'd come. While this sort of thing happens to everybody at some point, especially older folk, it had been happening to me four or five times a day.

Two years ago I had made up with my friend Andy Goldberg that I would pick up his seven-year-old daughter from town. I simply forgot to do it. Luckily, someone else covered for me, so there were no tragic consequences. But from that point forward, Andy wouldn't trust me with important things, and I could hardly blame him.

The other thing I had noticed about myself was that I no longer enjoyed setting up computer/Tech stuff the way I used to. I would buy something new and it would sit on the shelf for weeks before I would deal with it. I also kept trying to get my older son, Barak, to do it for me. I chalked this up to getting older. Older people tend to be technophobic, and I supposed that that was beginning to happen to me.

It took a new incident after I had already been diagnosed with MS to make me look into the cognitive issue.

I was in town when I got a call on my cell from Andy. He invited me to come over to his house to watch the Democratic debate. I was really glad to do this having not seen him in a while, and I look forward to watching the debate with someone so smart. (He is an Englishman who graduated from Cambridge.) I made up with him that I would go to my house first to help my wife Susie with a few things, and then I would come to his place.

I got home, I helped my wife, and I sat down to watch the debate.

I had no idea that I had forgotten about Andy until the following morning. Driving home from taking my son Zohar to school, I came to a fork in the road. One way would take me home; the other would take me to Andy's. It was only then that I realized that I had forgotten to watch the debates with him. This really scared me. I had so wanted to go! How could I have forgotten?

Back to the Internet for more research. Lots and lots of material on the cognitive impact of multiple sclerosis. Here's a quick summary from the national MS Society:

Cognitive Functions Affected in MS

In MS, certain functions are more likely to be affected than others:

   * *Memory (acquiring, retaining, and retrieving new information)*
   * *Attention and concentration (particularly divided attention)*
   * *Information processing (dealing with information gathered by the five senses)*
   * *Executive functions (planning and prioritizing)*
   * *Visuospatial functions (visual perception and constructional abilities)*
   * *Verbal fluency (word-finding)*

It seemed clear to me that my memory problems and inability to deal with tech was also a result of the MS. In fact, everything bad that it happened to me over the last eight years or so could be laid at the footsteps of multiple sclerosis.

The notion of degenerating into a blithering idiot appealed to me even less than the notion of ending up in a wheelchair. In fact it freaked me out. If I have any sense of personal identity, it's tied up with my intelligence. The thought of losing that made me understand the 15% suicide rate among MS patients a little better.

Once again, doing my own research, I discovered that there was a new drug called Provigil that helped keep one alert without the bad side effects of amphetamines. I got my doctor to prescribe it for me, and it has helped me a lot. Maybe a 50% improvement. I wasn't getting lost quite as often.

Unfortunately, my executive functions are not helped by the drug at all. My little boy had to help me assemble a new wagon I had bought for him. The five pages of instructions and the tens of screws, nuts and pieces brought my brain to a grinding halt.

Oh, Hell! How was I going to deal with this? My poor family. The last thing I wanted was to become was *"the sick man at home,"* a burden and a source of guilt for all of them.

2."God loves a cheerful man."

My father, Herman Wouk, at the age of 92 remains one of the smartest and sharpest people I have ever known. A deeply religious Orthodox Jew, he is also the closest person I have ever found to being a "Renaissance Man."

I remember when I was at Columbia College in 1972 I had gotten all involved with new left politics, in particular Students for a Democratic Society or SDS. I remember going home to visit my parents and spouting off in all directions about what was wrong with the country and the capitalist system that ran it.

The next time I came to visit, my father had re read Karl Marx et al and invited me into his office to discuss it. Needless to say he had a far greater grasp of the subject than I did. I came away with two different feelings. I was amazed and complimented by the fact that he had taken the time to do this. He was in the middle of writing *War and Remembrance* and had far more important things to concern himself with.

At the same time I was somewhat crushed and humiliated by his undeniable mastery of a subject for which I had the enthusiasm of youth and little more.

Thirty four years later, sitting out in the garden with him at his home in Palm Springs, I confided to him my fears of becoming a burden to all around me.

He acknowledged that what I was going through was extremely difficult, and that what ever I did to deal with it, it was going to be hard.

"There is one thing I have tried to remember when I'd gone through awful times. I don't know if this will help you. There is an old Jewish saying that 'God loves a cheerful man'." And then he added "And so does everyone else..."

I don't think a single phrase has ever affected me so much in my life. For the next two months I walked around with a smile on my face. I was nice and friendly to every body, including strangers, and to a man they returned those feelings and made me feel happy to be alive even with MS.

And yet... Eventually the hopelessness of my condition began to take its toll. I've never been one to accept defeat gracefully, and sitting around waiting under the sword of Damocles without an escape plan was something I couldn't tolerate.

About a month ago, I visited a friend of mine, Bob Forte. He was one of the first people we met when we moved to Santa Cruz, and is one of the larger figures in what's left of the psychedelic community. He was friendly with all the greats of the movement from Albert Hofmann to Timothy Leary to Terence McKenna.

I explained to him how frustrated I was that there didn't seem to be anything I could do to actually cure the MS. He looked thoughtful and then related to me stories about two people he knew who had been diagnosed with terminal cancer. One had melanoma, the other had breast cancer that had metastasized to her liver. With no hope left, both had opted to journey deep into the jungles of South America to a shaman there famous for miracle cures. He told me that both of them had returned completely healthy.

"Why don't I go with you down there? It might be your only shot at curing yourself. I think we could even write a good book about it..."

Bob has always believed in the great power of psychedelics to do good. He has written a number of books on the subject and was one of the first to use the term "enthiogen" to describe drugs that can give one a "religious experience."

For a period of about five years, which ended about 10 years ago, my wife and I had explored the psychedelic experience. At the time we noticed all sorts of magical things occurring including physical evidence left behind of what we had thought was a shared hallucination. But that was a long time ago. I had long since relapsed into my former, thoroughly rationalistic self. As the period of magic faded away, I managed to come up with rational explanations for most if not all of the magic. Bob on the other hand was still a believer.

"I'm sorry Bob, I just don't believe in miracle cures. If you don't believe in them, they don't happen."

"But that's the thing; Ayahuasca can affect your belief systems. One of the people I told you about was a college professor. About as rational a person as I know. I can put you in touch with her if you like..."

He had a point there I thought to myself remembering my magical period.

"Well, I've always thought that miracle cures whether brought about by the waters of Lourdes or shamanic magic are possible only because of the placebo effect. So what we're talking about doing is using psychedelics to *convince myself that I am cured...* This would hopefully engage the placebo effect to *really* cure me. Interesting…"

"So what do you think? I was planning on going down there in another few months anyway. You should come along. You might actually cure yourself and we might actually get a good book out of it."

I explained to Bob that the stress and strain of a trip to the jungle through the heat, bugs, and tropical diseases made it more than likely that I would suffer a relapse before I even got there. It's a well-known fact that heat, stress and physical exertion can bring about a relapse of MS.

"Maybe I can find a local shaman who can help. Just doing Ayahuasca won't work, I don't think. I will need the input of a real medicine man...."

Bob said he knew of some local shaman but that none of them could compare with the ones in the jungle. But, if I felt I couldn't handle the trip that might be the only way."

I decided I better do some serious research about the placebo effect. While I knew the effect was real and was a positive bother to the pharmaceutical companies when testing their drugs, I really didn't know how powerful the effect was in practice.

3. The Placebo Effect

Placebo effect is the term applied by medical science to the therapeutic and healing effects of inert medicines and/or ritualistic or faith healing practices. When referring to medicines, a placebo is a preparation which is pharmacologically inert but which may have a therapeutic effect based solely on the power of suggestion. It may be administered in any of the ways in which pharmaceutical products are administered.

Sometimes known as non-specific effects or subject-expectancy effects, a placebo effect (or its counterpart, the nocebo effect), occurs when a patient's symptoms are altered in some way (i.e., alleviated or exacerbated) by an otherwise inert treatment, due to the individual expecting or believing that it will work.

The placebo effect occurs when a patient takes an inert substance (sometimes called a "sugar pill") in conjunction with the suggestion from an authority figure or from acquired information that the pill will aid in healing and the patient's condition improves. This effect has been

known since the early 20th century. -
Wikipedia

Western medicine has to acknowledge the placebo effect, even though it is unable to understand the mechanism by which it works. The reason is simple; the placebo effect operates also when real medicines are administered. This causes a major problem when trying to analyze the effect of new drugs. Is the patient's improvement due to the activity of the drug, or due to the placebo effect?

That's why double-blind studies, where one group is given the active drug and the other given a non-active drug, are the only way to know if the active drug is worth anything. To give to you an idea of just how powerful the placebo effect is, if 24% of the people taking the active drugs improve and 20% of the people taking the placebo improve, this is considered a significant success for the active drug.

How well the placebo effect works depends on the whole variety of things. It is most effective for treatment of pain and other "subjective" symptoms, with success rates of 60 to 70%. Last month they released a study showing that placebos were equally as effective as Prozac and other SSRI drugs at fighting depression. As I mentioned before, Prozac pulled me out of the awful depression brought on by MS. If a placebo would've worked just as well, why wasn't that tried first?

The problem is, for Western medicine, the use of placebos to treat actual sickness raises all sorts of ethical problems. In order for the placebo to work the patient needs to believe that he is receiving real medicine. That means that the doctor is forced to essentially lie to his own patient. For obvious reasons that makes most doctors feel uncomfortable. Not only that, one could hardly blame a patient for suing a doctor for malpractice if he found out he was being "played" by the doctor rather than being "treated."

To give you an idea of how important it is that the patient "believes" that he is receiving a "real" drug, when doing double-blind studies the placebo administered is often an amphetamine, or vitamin B-12. This is in order to cause the patient to "feel" the drug, and thus believe he is in the group getting the active drug rather than the placebo. This apparently makes a big difference to how well the placebo effect works.

The various psychological explanations for how the placebo effect works are thoroughly inadequate. It has become clear that placebos can have a real physical effect on the body. It turns out those people given placebos to fight pain, when given a drug that blocks the effects of *opiates* have their pain return. This indicates that the *placebo effect caused the body to release endorphins*, the body's natural painkilling version of an opiate.

> *A "placebo response" can amplify, diminish, nullify, reverse or, even, divert the action of an "active" drug.*
>
> *Because a "placebo response" is just as significant in the case of an "active" drug as it is in the case of an "inert" dummy drug, the more that we can discover about the mechanisms that produce "placebo responses," the more that we can enhance their effectiveness and convert their potential efficacy into actual relief, healing and cure.*
>
> *Recent research strongly indicates that a "placebo response" is a complex psychobiological phenomenon, contingent upon the psychosocial context of the subject that may be due to a wide range of neurobiological mechanisms (with the specific response mechanism differing from circumstance to circumstance).*
>
> *The very existence of these "placebo responses" strongly suggest that "we must broaden our conception of the limits of endogenous human control"; and, in recent times, researchers in a number of different areas have demonstrated the presence of biological substrates, unique brain processes, and neurological*

correlates for the "placebo response." -
Wikipedia

Using pet scans and functional MRIs, the real, biological effects of placebos is beginning to be studied.

"Spontaneous remission" is how doctors describe it when someone gets better for reasons the doctor doesn't understand. This includes all "miracle cures" whether the result of the waters of Lourdes or the ayahuasca of a South American Shaman. In other words, spontaneous remission is simply a euphemism for Western sciences ignorance of how the body can heal itself, in cases where Western medicine is unable to help.

As a multiple sclerosis patient, my only hope for a cure is to somehow cause a spontaneous remission to occur. Who knows, if doctors were allowed to use placebos, maybe they could cure me with the placebo effect. But they aren't allowed to use them, so I can just forget about that.

What's a rationalist to do? The offerings of Christian Science and all the New Age Pyramids, crystals, magnets, herbs and what have you can't possibly work for me. I simply can't bring myself to believe in any of that stuff. Without belief -- no placebo effect. Without placebo effect -- no spontaneous remission.

The only chance I've got is to try to force myself to believe in the unbelievable. This is not easy for an agnostic, secular humanist like me. In fact it's impossible.

The only time I've ever believed in the unbelievable was as a result of psychedelics. It's amazing to me that the only chance I might have for a cure is completely illegal in this country. The decision to outlaw psychedelics back in the 60s was the result of a real fear on the part of the government at the time that the hippie movement would overwhelm them. Richard Nixon once actually said that Timothy Leary was "the most dangerous man in America."

Of course those fears are long behind us. The idea that psychedelics pose an addiction problem like the other hard drugs is absurd on its face. Psychedelics are self-limiting. The more often you use them the less well they work. Not only that, you don't take psychedelics to "feel good." As often as feeling good, they can scare the shit out of you.

In addition in order to get the effects of ayahuasca you have to be willing to endure real discomfort first. More often than not it makes people throw up with a vengeance and often gives them an extreme bout of diarrhea. Maybe that's why the Supreme Court recently allowed ayahuasca in the ceremonies of the Brazilian church that uses it. Before that the only legal psychedelics were peyote used in the ceremonies of the Native American Church. Guess what? Peyote also makes you puke…

I am a deeply law-abiding person. Both because I understand the necessity of having laws, as well as the desire to avoid the stress associated with the fear of getting caught.

But these drug laws, in addition not helping society, are standing in the way of my only chance to cure my multiple sclerosis. So screw them!

How dangerous would it be for me to take ayahuasca, whether here or down in South America? Checking on Medline this is what I found:

> *There was no evidence that ayahuasca has substantial or persistent abuse potential. Long-term psychological benefits have been documented when ayahuasca is used in a well-established social context. Conclusion A decoction of DMT and harmala alkaloids used in religious ceremonies has a safety margin comparable to codeine, mescaline or methadone. The dependence potential of oral DMT and the risk of sustained psychological disturbance are minimal.* - Addiction 2007 Jan; 102(1):24-34.

4. Zen and the Art of Multiple Sclerosis

What's Buddhism got to do with this?

On one level, nothing at all. The placebo effect? Amazonian shaman? Buddhism hasn't anything to do with either of them. But on a different level it speaks with the same voice.

Perhaps the most central concept in Buddhism is the fact and that everything in the universe relies on everything else in the universe in order to exist in itself.

One of the commonest hallucinations shared by many people who have taken ayahuasca is that of the Web. A web that connects everything in the universe with everything else in the universe. Ayahuasca forces you to see those connections. You see them as gray lines. Gray lines connecting everything to everything else.

This vision is precisely the same vision described as "Indra's net." Imagine a three dimensional spider's web. At every place where the webs intersect there is a jewel. Each jewel reflects all the other jewels. In each reflection in each jewel is contained the reflection of all the other jewels. Ad infinitum…

This underlying reality of Buddhism was labeled by Aldus Huxley as the "perennial philosophy." According to Huxley this is the same underlying reality that touched Christian saints as well as pagan shaman.

What it all comes down to is the realization that there is no way that one thing or event can exist with out every other thing or event - whenever it happened - for all time...

According to Buddhist philosophy, each one of us is "all there is" meaning "the entire universe" pretending it's just little old me.

In optics, an aperture is a hole or an opening through which light is admitted. The Buddhist view is that all conscious beings are apertures through which the universe views itself. The problem is that it is impossible to actually view that which is doing the viewing. Just as you can't see your eyes without a mirror, you can't see yourself as the whole universe.

Well, that certainly reinforces the notion that each of us has the power to cure ourselves. I mean, if we are everything, we ought to be able to fix something as simple as multiple sclerosis. Right?

I have been studying Buddhism, most specifically Zen, but all other variations as well for the last four years. My Guru is Alan Watts who has been dead since 1973. He would never have allowed me to call him a guru. Since he's dead, I'll do as I please.

The truth is I've never heard of Zen miracle cures.

Nevertheless, why not try for one? Is there any conceivable advantage in playing along with consensus reality this time? Consensus reality tells me there is no cure for my multiple sclerosis. The shaman holds out a potential cure. Even if the chances of it working are very small, it's better than anything else that's being offered.

Western society emphasizes the importance of the individual. By overdoing this, we have lost track of how we are connected to everything else in the universe. Balance is what is needed. We are individuals, and yet, we are all that there is.

Somehow shamanism seems to tap into this truth. "Wo.......!"

"What are you trying to tell me? That these primitives somehow know more truth than did Plato or Aristotle or Moses or Jesus or Einstein... gimme a break!"

The rationalist wakes out of his stupor...

"It's all crap! Crap made to seem like reality. Stop looking for false hopes! Accept the fact that you are screwed. Enough of this already..."

Despair...

Oh *to hell with you*, rationalist... I'd rather be cured than be intellectually honest. Or would I? I'm actually not sure...

Is a happy lie better than a painful truth?

"Damn the torpedoes.... I'll cure myself! Scientists and Doctors... Fair warning. Here comes another "*spontaneous remission*"!

5. What's quantum physics got to do with this?

Much like Buddhism, nothing and everything, depending upon the level one explores.

Despite the attempts to tie quantum physics to Eastern religion in books like, *The Tao of physics* or *The Dancing Wu Li Masters,* I have never run across an attempt to tie it in to Amazonian shamanism. I wouldn't imagine anyone would try to use quantum physics as a way of explaining the placebo effect either.

But at the same time quantum physics gives scientific proof to the notion that rationalism cannot always be used to explain reality. The kinds of truths that quantum physics asks us to believe go way beyond shamanism and placebo effects.

We are asked to believe that light, and everything else for that matter, is both a wave and a particle at the same time. Unless we look. When we look it resolve's itself into one or the other depending upon *how* we look i.e. the tests we run.

We are asked to believe that all the states of a particle can be either one way, or the other way or *both ways at once.* This is called being in a superposition, and is the basis on which quantum computers have been designed, built and actually demonstrated to work.

We are asked to believe in "entanglement" where two superpositioned particles, once related in a certain way, are able to instantly communicate their states one to the other even if they are a thousand light years apart. This was the "spooky action at a distance" as Einstein called it in his famous E.P.R. attack against quantum physics.

Because quantum physics resulted in such an absurd outcome, Einstein thought it proved something was missing from the theory. Instead, entanglement has since been tested in the laboratory, and been shown to actually happen. If Einstein had never deduced that the quantum theory implied entanglement, it might never been discovered. That's one of the reasons that scientists say Einstein *was right even when he was wrong.*

The other main reason was his "cosmological constant" that he introduced into his general theory of relativity in order to allow for a static universe. When Edwin Hubble proved that the universe was expanding, Einstein called his cosmological constant the biggest blunder he had ever made.

The recent discovery that the universe was not only expanding, but accelerating in its expansion, meant that the universe contained a repellent force as well as the attractive force of gravity. This was Einstein's cosmological constant brought back to life, and has been dubbed "dark energy" by cosmologists.

To return to entanglement, the implication of the theory is that everything in the universe is connected to everything else in the universe at instantaneous, superluminal speed. This is because at the "big bang" everything would have been entangled. Once entangled, always entangled. Sounds a bit like "Indra's net," no?

David Bohm tried to explain quantum weirdness with his implicate, explicate order theory. The universe exists on two levels, the explicate which we are all familiar with, and the implicate, which we can't see but which is there nonetheless.

The example often used to explain what is meant by "implicate" is what happens when you put ink drops in glycerin. The individual drops do not dissolve and they hold together as separate entities in the glycerin. Now, if you rotate the glycerin around and around the drops will fade out till they disappear.

When you rotate the glycerin in the other direction, the drops eventually reappear. The drops, originally explicate, become implicate in the rotation, and become explicate again in the counter rotation.

More "Indra's net" stuff. As I discussed in the previous chapter, Indra's net is closely related to one of the most common hallucinations on ayahuasca.

Sitting out on the grass with Bob, he asked me whether I thought my MS was somehow caused by myself or was just bad luck. You know, like being one of the ones Charlie Whitman picked off from his place in the university tower.

I told him I wasn't sure, but that the general feeling I got from the MS forums I visit was more the "bad luck" version. Here's what he responded.

"Look Joe, a lot depends on one's point of view and it is critical that you understand this. You know that light can manifest as either a particle or a wave depending upon which test you choose to run. I want you to consider the possibility that your sickness is being caused by something you have chosen during your life. The point is, that by looking at it that way it could actually *be* that way, the same way as in quantum physics."

Wow, that hit me hard… I sat and thought as deeply as I could. Everyone makes choices they afterwards regret. But I couldn't think of any at the moment. Until I came down with MS, my life had been almost literally "charmed." I mean that.

Best family, best schools, honorable Navy service in Israel, marriage to a brilliant actress/fashion model, two unbelievably wonderful sons, no real money troubles, living in the most beautiful place with the smartest and coolest people in the US… The list goes on and on.

It wasn't anything mentioned above, obviously. It had nothing to do with externals, they were all great. What about the internals? Was I comfortable with myself?

Was there any part of my life that bothered me? Something under the surface, a *hintergedagen* that could be manifesting itself through my MS?

Maybe…

The truth is that ever since the MS depression hit me 7 years ago I have basically been operating in "survival mode." Those readers who have ever been severely depressed should know what I'm talking about. I'll try to explain to those lucky enough not to know.

Essentially, "survival mode" the way I am using it refers to an intentional withdrawal from *anything* that could provoke a relapse of the depression.

I don't go to any movies that are sad or are violent. I avoid even thinking about tragedies, even when they're in the news. And I suppose I also avoid exposing myself to rejection.

That's where the problem could lie! I haven't written anything at all since the depression. I haven't traveled anywhere since the depression. I have had NO ambitions at all since the depression.

I used to explain my lack of ambition as a *positive* quality. A Taoist denial of the ego, if you will. But that always felt a little hollow to me.

Maybe I'm disgusted with myself for not having contributed much to anything or anyone for the last seven years.

Maybe? I *know* I feel that way, now that I think about it. It's just real hard to admit it.

So Bob wants me to view the MS as being caused by some self-inflicted injury. If it's anything, it's this. I will meditate on it and try to connect to whatever self-loathing I find. The point is not a psychological one. The point is to actually *change the reality* of my illness from a chance piece of bad luck to something I caused myself.

I know it sounds completely non-rationalistic. But the undeniable scientifically proven truth is that our choice of test *does* determine whether light manifests as a wave or a particle. Do we really know that our choice of attitude *can't* affect an illness?

Quite the contrary, placebos and spontaneous remissions *do occur.* Our internal attitude is critical in these effects. I will try my hardest to believe that I am causing this MS as a way of waking me out of the stupor of "survival mode."

Truth be told, it already has. My current word count on this book stands at 20,908. My posts to MS support forums of some of the chapters have been really appreciated by a lot of people. They like the content as well as enjoy my writing style. They tell me it makes them feel better to read it.

This makes me feel better than anything I have done since volunteering to fight for Israel after having completed Columbia Law School.

So maybe there is more of a quantum connection to this story than just proving rationalism to be limited.

Maybe…

It's just very hard to beat back the skeptic inside me.

6. What's DNA got to do with this?

Well, for starters, the scientists have figured out that multiple sclerosis has at least *some* genetic component. To give you an idea of how large a component; while the chance of getting MS in the population at large is about one in ten thousand, the chance of getting it if your sibling has it is three out of a hundred.

Big difference, no doubt, but it's not enough of a difference to conclude that MS is *caused* by faulty DNA, only that faulty DNA can be one element of multiple causes of the disease.

So there is a real connection between multiple sclerosis and DNA. We simply still don't understand what that connection is.

On the more "far out" side of things, a whole book has been written about the connection of the ayahuasca experience of shamans to DNA. In *The Cosmic Serpent: DNA & the Origins of Knowledge*, Jeremy Narby makes an argument that the structure of DNA has been known by primitives down through history. For proof he offers all sorts of coincidences involving snake or snake figures used as deities through history all over the world. He also draws on his personal experience using ayahuasca where he saw two silvery snakes.

> *I began my investigation with the enigma of "plant communication." I went on to accept the idea that hallucinations could be the source of verifiable information. And I ended up with a hypothesis suggesting that a human mind can communicate in defocalized consciousness with the global network of DNA-based life.*

All this contradicts principles of Western knowledge.

Nevertheless, my hypothesis is testable. A test would consist of seeing whether institutionally respected biologists could find bimolecular information in the hallucinatory world of ayahuasqueros... My hypothesis suggests that what scientists call DNA corresponds to the animate essences that shamans say communicate with them and animate all life forms. Modern biology, however, is founded on the notion that nature is not animated by intelligence and therefore cannot communicate. (page 132)

To sum up: My hypothesis is based on the idea that DNA in particular and nature in general are minded. (page 145)

When I first read the book when it came out in 1998, I was disappointed and found it utterly unconvincing. While the author piles on coincidence after coincidence through history, he fails to convince that there was anything more than coincidence behind them.

It's Robert Anton Wilson's "Rule of 23s," to wit, you always find what you are looking for when you look.

Ever notice when you get a new car that all of a sudden you start seeing the same make and model everywhere you look?

What Wilson did was claim that the number 23 had a special significance that we should all watch out for. It's an amazing experience when 23s seem to start popping up everywhere. The restaurant table number 23. My seat on the plane... Row 23. My friends address, 23 Elm st. , etc..... You get the idea.

What Wilson was trying to teach us was that our experience of reality is completely colored by what we bring to the table. Who ever noticed anything special about 23? Nobody. Not till Wilson mentioned it. And then it seemed unavoidable all around us!

So Narby found snakes, spirals, helixes etc. everywhere he looked. I would have been more amazed if he *hadn't* found them everywhere.

But now I was looking at the book through a different filter.

In the book Narby says, "After about a year in Quirishari, I had come to see that my hosts' practical sense was much more reliable in their environment than my academically informed understanding of reality. Their empirical knowledge was undeniable. However, their explanations concerning the origins of their knowledge were unbelievable to me."

That's to be expected. After all, Narby, holds a PhD in anthropology from Stanford University.

But boy did he change his tune after trying the ayahuasca himself!

> *After drinking ayahuasca, Narby had a profound life changing experience. His view on himself and reality shifted from an intellectually superior know-it-all to a mere human being that has no real understanding of reality at all. In his experience, these thoughts were telepathically imparted to him by two giant snakes.*

> The Vaults of Erowid

What difference does it make that I found his arguments unconvincing. What I believed wasn't the issue. He obviously believed it himself, profoundly and totally. So much so that he tried to prove it was true by writing a book.

If drinking ayahuasca could convince Narby of such a far-out theory, I have reason to hope that it will convince me that I am cured of MS.

If it convinces me as completely as it convinced Narby, who is to say that that might not be enough to engage the placebo effect and cure myself in objective reality as well?

Finally, another "coincidence" to toss onto the heap that Narby so carefully built.

According to the Associated Press, FRANCIS CRICK, the Nobel Prize-winning father of modern genetics, was under the influence of LSD when he first deduced the double-helix structure of DNA nearly 50 years ago.

7. Cognitive Hell

The date is April 9, 2008. I've just been through and am still experiencing my worst cognitive day. Maybe a lesion is growing on my frontal lobes. Jesus, I hope this book doesn't turn into the second half of *Flowers for Algernon.* But if it does, you'll be able to tell and can stop reading when and if it gets disjointed or simple-minded.

Aside from multiple room to room mental dislocations, for the first time ever I lost track of what I was doing in the middle of doing it.

That's not supposed to happen to even partially impaired folks, I think. I emailed my doctor and hope to hear from her tomorrow. I found an adult ADD info page online and sent it to her. Oh, by the way, my doctor is a Jewish black lesbian.

Let's hear it for Santa Cruz! I *really* love this town.

After the "watch on too tight" debacle, I pleaded with my father and got his help to hire a personal physician. Three thousand up front buys me the right to her help whenever I need it for whatever my insurance will pay her. Not that bad a deal when you consider the co-pays that I would end up spending, given my condition.

For those of you who have never experienced it, this is what cognitive decline feels like;

That's right. It "feels" like nothing at all. Think about it. How can one "feel" the absence of something? The only way he "feels" it is by knowing that he knows something even though he can't actually access the information. So when I walk purposefully into a room, I'm clued in that there's something I meant to do there. Even though I don't know what it is, I can usually reconstruct it by retracing my steps.

But what about the times I don't know that I know? In those cases there's no "feeling" at all. Life feels completely normal. It's only afterwards that the effects of my forgetting are felt by others and I am made aware of my memory loss.

When reminded like this, sometimes I completely remember, sometimes I "kinda" remember, as from a dream, and sometimes I am taken totally by surprise. "Huh? I said/did that? I don't remember. Why would I say/do that?"

But losing track of what you are doing while you are doing it, now *that's* scary.

What if it happens to me when I'm driving my son to school or fixing a shingle on the roof?

There is an old Jewish saying that I will transliterate for the tribe before translating.

Im lo ani li, me li?

"If I'm not for myself, who will be for me?"

It's getting harder and harder to be for myself. I am seriously losing self-confidence. At the moment the one thing I'm hanging onto is this book. Until I manage to try the ayahuasca shaman cure, it's like the only thing I *can* hang on to. Maybe that's because once I write it down, it stays. There's no way I can forget it if I chose to read it again.

I know that I promised to use humor and truth as my guides in writing this account. I'm sorry to say that truth most definitely has the ascendancy over humor this evening. I hope to make it up to you in later chapters. In general what I'm going through though, is ironic, and funny if also a bit painful.

Not this though. It feels like the Buddhist "void" coming to roost.

It feels like I'm looking in the mirror and watching myself dissolve, bit by bit, before my eyes.

8. *After the MRI*

As I suppose you could tell, I was beginning to panic when I wrote the previous chapter.

"Shit! What if I've got a new lesion growing on my frontal lobes? That wouldn't necessarily cause any physical symptoms, but it could show up in declining cognitive function."

My doctor got me into the MRI this morning. After taking a Valium, (I'm extremely claustrophobic) I spent my time relaxing and meditating as the huge machine whirred and pounded around my head for 45 minutes. No sweat. I've been through this four times before.

The first was the worst, of course. I had heard that I would be in a very enclosed place for a long time and I was nervous at the thought. Before going in, I smoked a fat joint, hoping that would relax me and get me through it.

What a mistake! Instead of relaxing me, it put me into a horrible paranoid place. Plus they had forgotten to give me the "emergency" bulb to squeeze if I needed out. I found myself shouting,

"Get me out of here! Help! Please....!"

We wasted a good ten minutes while they calmed me down, and then they gave me the bulb which I clenched to my chest like a magic talisman. Didn't need to use it, but somehow just knowing it was there made me relax some.

Today's results showed *no new or active lesions*. YAY! I'm slowly coming out of my anxiety state and refocusing on the task at hand, to wit, curing this disease.

I called my friend Bob Forte, and we agreed to meet out on West cliff beach. A few days earlier, we had agreed that he would play the role of Shaman to my role of patient. He told me that he had enough experience with ayahuasca that he could at least give it a try. As I mentioned earlier, I really wanted to try to give the experience a chance to work without having to go up a canoe for two days in the jungle.

Bob's taking his role very seriously. I think I would do the same in his position. He knows/believes that the ayahuasca is capable of healing, but it has to be done just right. I'm reminded of the wicked witch's line in *The Wizard of Oz* "These things must be handled d-e-l-i-c-a-t-l-y, or you spoil the spell..."

It's also his first chance to put into practice what he has learned over the years in his experiences with psychedelic (entheogenic) shamanism in order to effect a healing. When I thought about it, I realized that his helping me heal could make him feel even better than me. While he's not quite as old as I am, he's a pretty old soul. He figured out long ago that helping others always makes one feel better than helping oneself. It's weird how all these "tired" "hackneyed" truisms are brought into clear relief when dealing with things that *really* matter.

A week ago, he put me on a preparatory diet that avoids oils, white flour, and salt. For good measure, I also cut out meat and am trying to stick primarily to fresh organic vegetables. He also suggested plantains, but I've only got bananas which are similar if not identical. One is also supposed to avoid sex.

I'll go off the Prozac as well when the time gets closer. I'm afraid of going off it for too long, for obvious reasons. Once back in depression, I'm afraid the only visions I'll get from the ayahuasca will be fear and more fear. I'm expecting *some* fear, no matter what. But I'm beginning to get better at handling fear as every day goes by.

So today, Bob wanted to hammer some stuff into me that he thought I needed. The mind needs to be clear of preconceptions, ideas, plans, theories, and pretty much everything else for the ayahuasca doctor to be able to help.

Bob used the Buddhist metaphor of a clear pond of water. When it's windy, small waves and ripples are kicked up all over the surface and you can't see what's at the bottom.

On a quiet, still morning however, one can easily see to the bottom.

"That's where she is… On the bottom of the pond. You have to clear the choppiness out of your mind first to see her."

"Her?" I asked him quizzically. "Why 'her'? I've read all sorts of other accounts that involve…"

He cut me off mid-sentence. "Never mind all the other stuff you've read. My experience has been with a female presence and that's what I hope you'll experience."

OK by me, I thought. In general I don't associate femininity with fear. Of course there are always exceptions. The Hindu goddess Kali, for instance. She is generally pictured with blood dripping fangs. In one hand she holds a scimitar. In the other, the severed head of her husband, Shiva. The Hindus revere destruction as they do creativity. Each one requires the other to exist.

Bob focused on my old diet coke habit and my cigarette smoking. "You know both those things are bad, and yet you chose to do them. From the first time I met you 14 years ago, I knew that you were headed for health problems because of your self-destructive behavior."

I explained to him that as far as the coke went, I figured since they had been selling millions of cans every day for the last twenty years, that even if it wasn't particularly good for me, there were bigger things I should worry about. Once I found out about the MS I quit drinking it.

When I found out about the MS I also quit cigarettes for about a month. But given the strain and fear I was experienced every day, I decided to start again and at least have some antidote to misery I was in.

"I made the decision that even though smoking might seriously damage me in the future, I needed the comfort it gave me NOW. After all, we have to get through now before we even get to worry about the future."

He wasn't satisfied and accused me of "rationalization." How can I deny that when defending an addiction? "OK, so maybe all this is just an addict's excuses. All I can tell you is that I feel I need cigarettes now, and will not give them up. Maybe after the ayahuasca visions....

Bob then told me about a girlfriend of his who was an extreme nicotine addict and tossed them after one ayahuasca trip. Great! Maybe it will do the same for me.

Bob then began playing psychoanalyst. "Let's pretend for a minute that I'm some high paid shrink on the 20th floor of some building in Manhattan..."

"Are you out of your mind?! Why in god's name would you want to imagine that? LOOK for christsake..."

I waved my hand at the verdant spring vegetation exploding around us from all sides, the perfect clear blue sky, the Pacific Ocean crashing on the rocks below.

Bob laughed and beat a quick retreat, "Alright, let's just say that I'm a psychoanalyst sitting with you right here. I would begin digging around in your past searching for causes for your self destructive behavior, beginning with your father."

"That would be a waste of time," I told him. I've already sorted all those issues out long ago, both on my own and with psychedelic input." And I really have. All the childhood resentments that had carried over even into my 30s were long a thing of the past. I truly love both my parents without reservation, warts and all.

"Yes, he said, but you can't deny that your problems, neuroses and self destructive behavior must have originated somewhere in your past?"

I thought about this for a minute and then I answered, "Bob, one of the most useful things I've learned from Buddhism is that blaming the past for your present situation is an illusion. There *is* no past. There *is* only now. It's the NOW that affects the past, such as it is. Think about forgiving someone who has hurt you. When you do that, you change the *meaning* of the past.

What is the past, when you come right down to it? All it is is your memories of 'presents' gone by. While your memories may affect choices you make, you are free to ignore them and start anew. Think of it like this; the present is like a ship slicing through the water. The past is like the wake it leaves behind it. You're at the wheel of the ship and can change directions regardless of the wake."

I explained that I had left the past behind me where it belonged. That included all supposed injuries inflicted on me, whether by my parents or anyone else.

Bob liked my ship analogy. I could tell he was still unsure about me, though. He suggested that maybe I should take some meditation lessons. I told him that I had been using meditation ever since suffering from panic attacks at the early, undiagnosed phase of MS. I had picked up a book with a title something like, "*Meditation for Skeptics Who Believe Nothing.*" That title described me to a "T" so I bought the book and gave it a try.

People who don't know better think that meditation is some sort of spiritual experience where you connect somehow with "*the which than which there is no whicher.*" If you meditate looking for that, you'll get nowhere and quit. What meditation is is a method to quiet your mind so that you can actually experience reality as it is. Not what you project; hope, fear, whatever. What really *IS*.

There are a number of techniques for accomplishing this "still the mind" goal. The one I was taught both by our marriage counselor and by the little book above was simply to count your breathing. Up till four, then start over. If you lose track of where you are, just start over. When you find thoughts intruding, don't worry about it. Just start counting again. That's all there is to it, believe it or not…

I found that when I did it, it always calmed me down. Sometimes I would actually even feel refreshed afterwards.

But Bob thinks I could use some more techniques. He says you can accomplish more that way. OK, sure. I'll go where he tells me. My only problem with meditating is that sometimes I just can't relax and get bored as hell. Maybe that's why I've always avoided group meditation.

"Yikes! What if I get trapped for an hour of endless boredom?" But truthfully, that has rarely, if ever happened. I actually had a pretty good time back in the pounding MRI, now that I think of it.

I know that I am ready for the ayahuasca. I've been working towards it for well over a month. I know that my mind is open to accept whatever comes down the pike. I also know that I won't get anywhere if I go into the experience expecting and demanding a cure.

No. I will do my best to be joyous and receptive to whatever happens. And Bob will be there with me. And he really loves me.

It might even have a *better* chance of working than with an Amazonian shaman who doesn't know me and doesn't speak English.

Maybe that's just another wish-fulfilling rationalization on my part to avoid going to the jungle. But I don't think so. I'm a great believer in the power of friendship.

Besides, as I told Bob today, I've made up my mind. If we make no headway here, I *will* go with him to the jungle. If it gives me a relapse, so be it. I *have* to try to cure this MS. And if I can't, maybe I can find a way to true peace anyway.

Uh, oh…. As I mentioned earlier, "hope springing eternal" had gotten me into trouble time after time again.

But when you come right down to it, what else is there?

9. Footprints of God

Over the last ten years or so, I have been involved in reading just about every science book I could get my hands on. It began with a book called *The Arrow of Time*. I remember, at the time, being blown away by how little science really could tell us about time. What it really is and why it is unidirectional. Apparently, all the formulas that science uses regarding time can be run in the opposite direction as well, and there's great dispute over why, in reality, they can only be run forward.

I mean, if the passage of time isn't understood, what is? So I picked up a copy of *The Cosmic Code* by Pagels. Another revelation. Quantum physics remains the most impossible to understand truth that we seemed to have discovered. This laid the groundwork for what was to follow.

Physics, biology, genetics, chaos, information theory, complexity, emergence… The list goes on and on. I would read each book and have a wonderful feeling afterwards that I understood *more*.

I came to the conclusion that what I had been looking for all these years or at least what had been motivating me was a sense that science seems to run into walls no matter which direction is chosen. Ultimately, all our measurements seem to turn into *Cantor Dust* when we take them out to their logical extreme. No ultimate answers. In any direction. Ever.

I might as well try to define *Cantor Dust* as I believe it is extremely useful in demonstrating what it is that I am trying to describe overall.

Here's a quick rundown on Cantor Dust….

"For the Cantor dust example, we start with a large segment (the initiator), divide it in three equal smaller segments, and take out the middle one. This process (the generator) repeats indefinitely, producing the cantor dust." [1] The "dust" consists of an *infinite number of segments whose total length amounts to ZERO.*

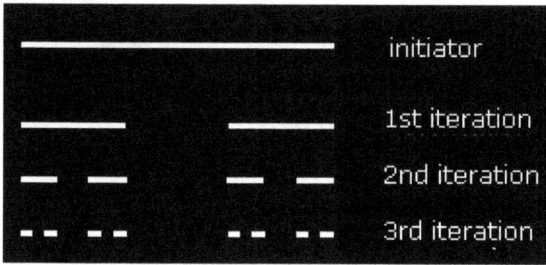

Thus was born the working title for a book I thought of writing, *Footprints of God.* The idea is that "God" (used here as a shorthand for the indefinable) has left its footprints behind on reality.

These footprints manifest as *impenetrable barriers to the scientific explanation and understanding of reality.* When I say impenetrable, I mean as defined by our best current theories of science. In other words, our science recognizes these barriers and is the source of their definition.

Quantum Physics

Of course the most obvious examples lie in Quantum Physics. Often described as one of, if not *the* most tested and validated theory in the history of science, quantum physics uses mathematical formulas to predict statistical outcomes of sub-atomic particle events. It works. Always.

The problem is in translating the math into concepts we can grasp. We can't. All the various interpretations lead to conclusions that simply make no sense to us. Particles are both particle *and* waves. Or one or the other, depending upon which test we run.

Bell's theorem shows that faster-than-light information can be transmitted unlimited distance. A particle linked to another particle then moved to the other side of the galaxy will cause the other particle to set its spin direction when its spin is measured.

---

[1] From *The Nature of Fractals*, http://www.fractovia.org/what/what_ing1.shtml.

Classic monstrosities like Schrödinger's Cat remain unanswered. The more we know about a particle's location, the less we *can* know about its direction. And what is the meaning of "measurement" anyway. Doe's this involve human consciousness in the actual *creation* of reality? Lots of people believe it does… It goes on and on like this.

Relativity

Einstein didn't like the "dice throwing" involved with quantum physics, though he was one of its central creators. He is much better known for giving us relativity, both Special and General. E=mc2 is actually his way of telling us that matter, i.e. *stuff* is actually energy. A whole hell of a lot of it! Mass multiplied by the speed of light squared. (Approximately 300,000 kilometers per second!) Fine.

Except that his relativity theories left us with all sorts of things we can't really comprehend as well. It predicted black holes… *singularities* where the laws of physics as we understand them *cannot* apply. What does apply in their place? By definition *we can't know*.

And guess what? Hubble telescope has been turning up all sorts of evidence of black holes out there. So according to Einstein, our immutable laws of physics apply only to *part* of the universe.

Perhaps the most famous wall we can attribute to Einstein is the speed of light itself. According to the theory, matter cannot move faster than the speed of light. The universe has a speed limit. What happens is that the closer and closer matter moves to the speed of light, the more and more mass it acquires, (the more it weighs) until at the end point, matter moving at the speed of light will have *infinite mass.* That's not possible, right?

Or is it? Black holes have infinite mass, by the same theory. Would moving matter at the speed of light just create another kind of singularity?

Life

We've been celebrating the decoding of the human genome for the last few years. Amazing piece of work! We're engineering rats that glow green and goats that produce spider web material in their milk. Only a question of time till we get to the bottom of this problem and start *creating* life forms from scratch, right? Nope.

Putting aside the issue of the thousands of proteins created by each of the thousands of genes, we're really no closer to understanding what makes things alive than we were in biblical times. Hard to believe, but there it is. We see how life is made up of chemical combinations of molecules. We have *no idea* whatsoever what it is that causes these molecular combinations to *live*.

Anyone who tries to identify what it is ends up creating a "black box" with some made-up term.

Perhaps the most famous of these black boxes is *Vitalism* which has been loudly put down by all reasonable scientists, but which remains the only modern attempt to explain life.

Complexity and Emergence

The newest "black box" to emerge, (heh!) is *emergence*. This is the word used to describe the fact that in nature, the sum is often more than the parts. Break the human body down into its chemical components and you'll get an idea what that means.

The notion is that once a certain level of complexity is reached in a system, new structures, unrelated to the structures of the components, "emerge" out of the sum of the components.

The problem is that by their very nature, complex systems cannot be predicted. The very best anyone hopes for once this "science" matures is to be able to predict possibilities.

Although I am unaware at this point of any scientific theory that proves we can never penetrate this mystery, all indications are and have been, that it is indeed impenetrable. Another footprint.

All these "footprints" show us the limits of Rationalism as a method of finding truth. But the ultimate proof of the limits of Rationalism is known as *Gödel's Incompleteness Theorem.*

10. Gödel's Incompleteness Theorem

At the risk of losing my audience, I wanted to cover this topic because I feel it underlies my justification for trying to cure my MS in an *irrational* way. If you start to haze over reading it, please just skip to the next chapter. While I try to explain it in a way that anyone can understand, I'm not sure how good a job I've done. I'm actually not sure that a good job *can* be done…

Gödel's Incompleteness Theorem is the granddaddy of them all, since it applies to mathematics which lies at the very *core* of all science. One could safely call mathematics the ultimate Aristotelian "First Philosophy" because it is basic to *all* science before one adds the particular details of any one science.

Gödel showed that within a rigidly logical system, propositions can be formulated that are undecidable or indemonstrable within the axioms of the system. That is, within the system, there exist certain clear-cut statements that can neither be proved nor disproved.

Hence one cannot, using the usual methods, be certain that the axioms of arithmetic will not lead to contradictions … It appears to foredoom hope of mathematical certitude through use of the obvious methods.

Perhaps doomed also, as a result, is the ideal of science - to devise a set of axioms from which all phenomena of the external world can be deduced.

Thus, Rationalism is by nature self-limited and unable to explain everything that happens to us in the world.

The bottom line is that Gödel's incompleteness theorem gives me *a rational basis to abandon Rationalism* as my only source to seek a cure for this multiple sclerosis.

Why does this matter to me? It matters because of the subtitle of this book, "*A Rationalist Seeks a Miracle Cure.*" While that might appear to be *self-contradictory* at first, Gödel gives it meaning again.

I remain a rationalist, even though I acknowledge that Rationalism is self-limiting. Rationalism is still the best system ever devised for finding truth. It simply is incomplete, i.e. some truths *must* be found outside it.

Here's *Gödel's* proof in plain English:

1. Suppose we have a **COMPUTER** supposedly capable of correctly answering any question.
2. Now consider the following proposition:

> **"The COMPUTER will never say that this sentence is true."**

1. Now, what happens when we ask the COMPUTER whether that proposition is true?
2. If COMPUTER says it is true, then "*COMPUTER will never say this sentence is true*" is false.

3. If "*COMPUTER will never say that this sentence is true*" is false, then the proposition is false (since proposition = "*COMPUTER will never say G is true*").
4. So if COMPUTER says the proposition is true, then the proposition is in fact false, and COMPUTER has made a false statement.
5. So COMPUTER will never say that the proposition is true, since COMPUTER makes only true statements.
6. We have established that COMPUTER will never say the proposition is true.
7. So "*COMPUTER will never say the proposition is true*" is in fact true.
8. So the proposition is true (since the proposition = "*COMPUTER will never say that this sentence is true*").
9. We have thus produced a true statement which COMPUTER cannot make.

Therefore...

That ayahuasca may cure my MS, could well be a truth which Rationalism cannot support. However, what matters ultimately, is the truth. Not the method by which we arrive at it.

Bob thinks I have a neurotic and incorrect view of the meaning of Rationalism.

While I may indeed be neurotic, I think I understand rationalism about as well as it *can* be understood. Warts and all, it's still the best system we've got. It's just that it has failed me in this particular case. Gödel makes it possible for me to accept this.

11. What's Meditation Got to Do With This?

"Wait a minute; didn't we have a whole chapter on Buddhism already? What's the idea?" I hear you cry…

Well, to make it as clear as I can, meditation is to Buddhism what a delicious meal is to a great cookbook. In other words, Buddhist philosophy is one thing, Buddhist practice another.

This chapter will try to lay out what I think about Buddhist practice, and how I think it might help my MS and/or me as a person.

I've already mentioned how easy it is to meditate. Just count your breaths etc. But what is it that we get out of the experience? What's the point?

If I were a Zen master I might answer with something like…

"The spring flowers have burst forth, some short, some long…"

Huh???

The thing is, the master can't answer properly using words, so he uses metaphors.

Alan Watts said that the purpose of poetry is to "*say what can't be said.*" That's what your question to the master requested, so he does the best he can.

The point is you don't "get anything" out of meditation. Meditation is a technique that allows your brain to see past the cultural models that each brain develops as it grows from childhood back to the raw sensory data that underlies it.

An example I like to use that most people can connect with is as follows:

Have you ever gone to sleep in a strange place? You know, a friends house or a hotel. And then, when you *first* wake up and open your eyes all you can make out is a bunch of unfamiliar shapes. Then, as your consciousness gets a little stronger, the model building part of your mind kicks in and…WHOOOOM!!! You are in a bed. And the bed is at your friend's house.

OK. Now try to imagine doing that in reverse and you'll get an idea of what meditation can do for you. The biggest difference, though, is that you are in a state of alertness rather than coming off sleep.

What's it "feel" like? Well I'm no Zen master so I can try to describe it to you as best I can. But trust me; you truly won't have an idea of what it's like from my words. There's a reason that the experience is called "ineffable," and it isn't to make it sound profound or important. It's because it's an "experience" and words simply can't describe a subjective experience.

That may sound like an outrageous overstatement to some, but at least let me explain what I mean first.

It doesn't matter which experience you choose. I will choose happiness as my example, if you don't mind. Alright, try to define happiness without using the word happiness or a synonym.

I'm serious, try to do it now…..

Hmmmmmm………….

That's right, you can't! But we don't need to. Since we are similar organisms we are able to label experiences that all of us share with words. If you tell me you are happy, I just remember being happy myself, and so I understand you. That's not the same as describing it. The truth is that not just meditation, but ALL experience is ineffable.

So in order to really know what meditation feels like, you simply have to do it. Once you have done it you can talk to other meditators and speak in a way that would make absolutely no sense to a non-meditator.

OK. With that behind me I will try my best to tell you what happened to me today in my first ever, public meditation session.

Everything I describe here is merely my own subjective experience. Bob seemed to indicate to me when I described it, that he knew what I was talking about, so maybe it is common.

When I first sit, I have to find something that I can focus on continuously. My first attempt today was to focus on a candle flame in front of the Buddha statue. I stared and counted my breaths. Something wasn't working. Maybe because the flame was moving, I don't know. I looked around for something else to fixate on.

Next to the leader was a white Kleenex box that stood out. I focused first on the box, and then narrowed my focus to a flower decoration on it. Counting my breaths, it began to happen...

Peripheral vision, what Alan Watts calls the "floodlight" rather than the focused "spotlight" of consciousness begins to do its thing. In my case, it was quite psychedelic. A bright yellow halo surrounded every blue pillow in the room. The floor, which was wood, began to change color in a wave, from grayish to bright and back again over and over.

And then I thought, "This is cool!" and *instantaneously* I was back in the consensus version of reality. By thinking "this is cool" I began model building in my mind, and so I was right back where I started.

What I try to accomplish when I meditate is to deconstruct the models I build in my brain and just experience what IS. The psychologists refer to the "oceanic" feeling that a newborn infant has. No model building at all. As a result, it's all one experience. You and everything around you are one experience.

Sadly we can't remember what it felt like to be an infant, but a successful meditation session will give you an idea.

Very good, but what's any of this got to do with multiple sclerosis.

I'm not sure, but Bob is. He explained it to me thus: "Your operating system, that which controls the whole organism, is out of whack. The trick is to access those parts that are wrong and fix them. In order to do that, you have to empty your cup."

Bob was referring to the Zen tale where a University Professor seeking wisdom from a master sits with him for tea. The master fills his cup then continues filling so that the hot tea overflows. The visitor jumps up, "Master, why?"

The master responds, you ask me to teach you Zen. Your mind is so filled with conceptions that it has no space. If you want new tea, you must first empty your cup. Only then, can you fill it again.

He spoke of a wonderful Buddhist concept I had never heard of before called prapancha which roughly means over conceptualizing things to death. I guess kind of like what I'm doing in this book.

Sigh!

I can't help myself; I just love it too much.

Lao Tzu starts the Toa Te Jing with the phrase:

> *The Tao that can be spoken is not the true Tao…*

And yet Lao Tzu *said* that. He couldn't help himself either. It's part of our nature to conceptualize, and there's nothing wrong with it. What's wrong is mistaking your conceptualizations for reality. And I gave you fair warning at the start of this chapter that what you would read would not really tell you that much. That's exactly what Lao Tzu was doing.

In any event, I told Bob that my cup was already pretty clean and that I had tried to toss all the cultural and personal models out.

"Do you understand the role you play in creating reality?" He peered at me as a wave crashed thirty feet below us on the rocks.

"Let's get something straight." I answered. "I don't exist. Not in the sense that there is something other than the organism itself that is "me" riding around in it. There *is* no homunculus inside us. All I am is an image that I carry around in my memory based on past experiences and on the reactions of others to me. And that image has to be as distorted an image as can exist, albeit the most complete. It has no deeper ontological reality than any of my other 'thoughts…'"

Bob waved me down, "I'm not talking about that, I'm talking about the WHOLE you….Hey, look, a WHALE!" he shouted..

Out about 200 feet from our perch on the cliff we watched as the great beast rolled past us, spouting as he went.

"Of course I understand the role I play. I'm all there is. I mean all my experiences result from my consciousness; there is nothing else to experience."

Bob nodded and looked out to see if the whale would resurface. "You told me that when we meditated, occasionally philosophical thoughts would intrude and you would catch yourself and refocus on the flower and the breathing."

"Yes. Not only philosophical thoughts, but also thoughts of how I might describe the experience in my book."

"Did you notice how or why those thoughts arose?"

I thought about this for a minute. It's always so hard to keep track of what your mind does. "I can't really say. The thoughts just drift in. The same way those waves crash on the rocks below. There's really no difference. It's all 'Ta ta ta…'" I used the Buddhist expression that means roughly, "reality, the way it is, all happening at once."

"Do you know what a mind moment is?"

I admitted that I had never heard the term before.

Bob turned to face me and then slapped his hands together. Whack!

"What the Buda teaches is that there are a trillion 'mind moments' in the course of that clap."

Of course I knew he was right. A long time ago I had had the experience of one night feeling as long as six months while on LSD.

"OK. Got you. Why do you bring that up?"

"As you progress in your meditation you will ultimately see how and where the thoughts come from as they intrude on you. It's really a question of mindfulness more than anything else. What you want to do is to experience those trillion mind moments."

"What's this got to do with the ayahuasca," I asked. "It sounds cool, but I'm not sure where you're going with it."

Bob smiled. "Don't you see? That's the kind of attention the ayahuasca healer can give to you."

"So?"

"So you're going to find out what's gone wrong with your operating system. Just like in psychoanalysis, once you find out the cause the symptoms can go away. All by themselves…"

12. *"Where the hell am I?!!!"*

Took a day off from writing yesterday. I couldn't write. All afternoon I busied myself with blogging, news, internet porn, listening to physics lectures. ANYTHING that would distract me from thinking. I was alone at home and began calling anyone I could think of for support, starting with my doctor.

"What's up, Joe?" She asked in her usual easy going manner.

"Hi Grace. Listen, I'm not sure if I'm calling you just for reassurance or whether it's something, as my doctor, you should know…"

What I told her was that on my way home from visiting with my friends Steve and Ellen, taking the same route I've been down hundreds if not thousands of times before, I suddenly had no idea where I was, where I was going, where I had come from…

I'm not sure if I knew who I was, but I might have since I realized I was having an "episode" and didn't panic but tried to figure out what had so suddenly vanished. I looked around and recognized nothing. I kept driving and looking at the street signs. No help there, I didn't recognize them. I figured if I just kept driving straight I would eventually see something I recognized.

Sure enough, about four or five blocks later I came to Ocean Street, which is one of the main streets in Santa Cruz. Got it! So I'm going in this direction across Ocean… That means I'm on my way home… Right! And I was at Steve's house before. Got it!

And I was back. Back, in the usual movie that each one of us creates in our minds. You know the one you always star in every morning till sleep time. Sometimes in dreams as well. What is it that gives it the feeling of a movie? Continuity. There's a system in our consciousness that stitches events in time together to form a narrative of sorts of our experience. I think it's that system that the MS occasionally interferes with.

A very weird experience. It felt as if someone had taken a scissors and cut the movie.

"What the?.....Where the hell am I?!!!"

It didn't last very long. Maybe 30 seconds or so. And I recovered and even remembered to drop something off for my wife in town before going home. I was proud that I didn't forget to do that.

But once I got home, things changed for me. I thought about the experience and began building all sorts of fantasies as to where this disease was taking me. None of them good.

I got caught in a "fear loop" that whirled round and round getting scarier with each revolution.

"What if next time it lasts 30 minutes?" "What if next time I won't recognize Ocean Street." "What if next time I forget how to drive?" On and on and on…

I took two valiums and got into bed to wait for my wife and son to come home. At this point I felt emotionally almost paralyzed. "Maybe I'm overdoing this?" I thought to myself. "Maybe NOT too…"

Once again it's important to point out that this experience doesn't "feel" like anything. If I hadn't been driving, just walking, I might not have even noticed. That's what makes the whole thing so frightening. You don't really know that it is happening till afterwards. And then it makes no sense.

I mean, why did I lose it there and then? I thought back over everything that had happened before. I was looking for any sign of a cause/ effect, if you will. The only thing I could come up with was that I hadn't taken my second Provogil of the day which I usually have at noon. The episode happened around 1:30. But that didn't really make any sense. The single Provogil works all day, the second is more a booster to keep me going past 5 PM.

After I called the doctor I called my father. He had trouble understanding what it was that I had experienced. That's when I came up with the metaphor of the film being cut.

"Now you listen to me," he said with as authoritative a tone as he could muster, "Write that down!"

"I can't. Not now. I'm in bed." I explained.

My dad went on, "Alright but be sure you include that in your book. That's an amazing description that gets the idea across beautifully. Your mind is more than fine, it's superb. You have nothing to worry about, OK?"

"Thanks Pop. Coming from you, that means a lot. You are after all, the master of words."

After I hung up I was left with the question of how it was possible to express myself in a way that even *dad* thought was good while at the same time not knowing where I was.

Sometimes when speaking, I just can't come up with a word, even a common one. I wave my hand and point to my head, "Mad Cow!" Usually I can get the word after grinding for 10-30 seconds, but not always.
I know now that I have gotten completely garrulous and so usually preface any long remark by asking if I had told my audience this before. More often than not, I have.

That's another nice thing about writing. As long as you read what you've written, you don't tend to repeat yourself.

What sort of a "cure" am I looking for from the ayahuasca? Do I seek to simply stop any more relapses or do I hope to get my mind back?

Sigh!

As I've said before, when it comes to health, hope springs eternal.

13. Lights in the Rear View Mirror

This is a crazy party I'm at. It's going on in three or four weird houses all of which have strange connecting passages and stairs from room to room and floor to floor.

There are pillows on the floor and people everywhere milling about and somehow I've lost track of my wife. I start calling "Suzie... Suzie!" No answer. People are looking at me like I'm nuts.

I start searching everywhere. Up and down twisted stairways, one room after another... One house after another. At one point I notice a room off to the side where I can see a couple on a bed making love. It's like Burning Man in the city.

"Have any of you seen my wife?" I plead with a group of revelers. One answers that they saw her a little while ago, but don't know where she is now.

"Suzie!" I keep yelling, hoping somehow she'll hear me over the din of electronic music which seems to be everywhere.

"Has she run off with someone?" I think to myself. This is it! I've HAD it.

Somehow I finally find her. "Suzie! I've been looking everywhere for you. Where have you been?"

She shrugs and goes back to talking to whoever she was talking to. My fury and anguish rise inside me and I yell, "All right, if that's how you want it we'll get a divorce..."

She looks at me coolly, shrugs again like she couldn't care less, and goes back to her business.

"Arrrrrgh!" I lunge to try to grab her by the throat and squeeze it until she *does* gives a shit.

And then I wake up….

Oh thank god! Just a nightmare. OK, I can deal with that. It'll be OK. She's right next to me in bed. I wake her and quickly tell her about the dream. "Poor baby," she says, "I'm sorry…"

I can tell that she means it, and I begin to calm down from the "fight or flight" chemicals coursing through my body.

And then, as consensus reality begins to get a better hold on my consciousness, I begin to run the movie of my life through my head to locate where I am in it. I know I'm supposed to drive my youngest son to school this morning, and thinking of that cues me in to what happened to me yesterday.

The HORROR! I wished I was back in my nightmare…

Here's what had happened:

Returning on a 7 AM flight from Palm Springs where we spent Passover with my parents, we had dropped Zohar off at school directly from the airport before going home. Suz was completely exhausted and needed to nap, so I volunteered to pick him up after school and take him to his special-ed dyslexia class from 5 to 6 PM.

I needed to leave at 4 because his school is in Aptos, a 45 minute drive from Bonny Doon where we live. I said goodbye to my older son, Barak, and asked him if we needed anything from town. He said we were out of bread, and I said I would stop and get some.

I got into the car and set up my Iphone in the holder which was hanging from the vent on the passenger side of the dash. I thought about moving it to the vent in front of me and then dismissed it. What difference did it make?

I drove down the winding mountain road to get to highway 1 which would take me through Santa Cruz and then off to Aptos. As usual, I was listening to NPR which had the 4 PM news going. By the time I got to the highway, the main news had finished and they were beginning a program that always bored me. I decided to switch to my Iphone and listen to an Alan Watts lecture on Buddhism.

I was speeding up to 55 which is the speed limit. I always use cruise control to make sure that I don't exceed the limit through inattention. As I accelerated I leaned over to press the "play button" to start the lecture. It didn't work at first, and I had to press it a few times to get it to play. Then I noticed that I had swerved across the yellow divider while my attention had been on the Iphone. I instantly corrected it and checked my speedometer at the same time. I saw I was still only at 45 mph, so I accelerated to 55 and set the cruise control.

Then I checked my rear view mirror and saw a cop car with lights flashing behind me.

"He probably needs to pass me," I thought to myself and so hit the brake and pulled over to the curb to let him get by. Instead of passing, he pulled behind me. "Oh shit," I thought, "He's after me. But why?" I brought the car to a halt. I could hear him saying something from a loudspeaker, but couldn't make out what it was, so I rolled down my window.

A mechanical sounding voice was saying, "Drive down to the next road and turn off…"

I began to do as instructed, all the while wondering what I possibly could have done to make him want to pull me over. Then I remembered how I had swerved when fussing with the Iphone. That must be it. SHIT!

The truth of the matter is I try to drive like a frightened grandmother these days. I take NO chances anymore. The days of radar detectors to beat speed limits were way behind me. As were rolling stops, ignoring meaningless stop signs in the middle of nowhere, etc. All the usual shortcuts that a lot of us are guilty of all the time. I DON'T DO THAT ANYMORE. And here I was getting pulled over anyway.

A young, handsome police officer came up to my car and I handed him my license. "I'm sorry, I was trying to get my Iphone to play and I somehow lost track of the road and swerved," I explained.

"Yes, the swerving is one of the reasons I stopped you, but at one point you were also going 80 miles an hour." He answered.

I blanched, "80?!!!! I thought I was going 45!"

"Have you been drinking?"

"I don't drink," I answered.

"Wait here," he nodded and went back to his car to run my license.

I slumped over the wheel in absolute terror. If I was really going 80 when I thought it was 45 then my cognitive problems had reached a new low. Trembling and breathing hard I tried to think what I should do.

If he wanted to test me for drinking, I knew I would fail the "walking a straight line" test. My balance has been off enough since I was diagnosed with MS that I knew I was incapable of passing it. I decided I would ask to blow up the balloon, instead. That at least would prove I had no alcohol in my body.

The cop came back with his ticket writing folder in his hand.

"Was I really going 80?" I looked at him with pleading in my eyes.

"I'm not exactly sure, I didn't have the radar on, but you were definitely somewhere in that neighborhood."

"You don't understand," I said. "I have multiple sclerosis. Last week I was driving through the middle of town and suddenly had no idea where I was."

"Really?" he said. I could see a look of worry cross his face. "Did you see me coming at you when you swerved?"

I searched my memory of the event. "I remember swerving. I don't think I saw any car. Certainly not a POLICE car! I don't think I could have possibly ignored that if I had seen it."

I continued, stammering, "You have to understand, the point is, if I was going 80 when I thought I was going 45 then I'm worried about driving at all. I mean I could be a REAL menace... Please, tell my wife what happened... Please!" I pleaded with him as I dialed home on the Iphone.

Suz picked right up. I guessed she had already woken from her nap.

"Suz, listen. I got pulled over by a cop. He says I was going 80 when I thought I was going 45." My voice was trembling, on the verge of hysterical. "Please talk to the officer; I don't know what to do."

I handed the Iphone to the cop who spoke with Suzie. "Well, I only wrote him up for crossing the line, but now he's not feeling comfortable about continuing on to pick up your son."

He handed the phone back to me, went back to his car and drove off.

Suz said she didn't think I should drive at all, that she would come pick me up.

"No. Forget it. I know I can make it home. I'm only a mile or so down highway 1. You've got to go get Zohar, or get a friend to pick him up. I'm way too shook up to make it to Aptos and back..." Aptos is a 50 mile round trip from our house.

"Alright," she said in a soothing voice. "Come home. I'll deal with Zohar, don't worry."

Hanging up, I wondered if I had made a mistake. After all, if I couldn't tell I was going 80, maybe I might miss a mountain curve and go over a cliff. I thought about calling her back and asking to be picked up.

I sat in the car for maybe five minutes flipping and flopping as to what was the right thing to do. I mean it wasn't only me that could be hurt/killed if I zoned out again.

In the end I decided to give it a try... REAL slow, so that even if I had an "episode" I was unlikely to hurt anyone. There's almost no traffic at all going up the hill and I figured I could make it the mile or so down the highway to the turn off.

Obviously I did make it home, since I'm now writing this.

"What happened?!" Suzy demanded the second I walked into our bedroom.

"I don't know," I answered, "The best I can do is telling you my version of it as I remember. Barak!" I called my 18 year old son to come hear as well. I now rely on him almost as much as I do on my wife.

I related the whole story to them as best as I could.

"That cop was lying," Suzy said. "He obviously thought you were drunk when he saw you swerve. He was going to try to bring you down with everything he could come up with..."

"I agree," Barak said, shaking his head. "Think about it. If you were really going 80, why didn't he write you up for it?"

"He said his radar wasn't on," I answered. "Maybe he thought he didn't have the evidence to prove it."

"That's ridiculous," Barak continued. "Wasn't he driving behind you for a while before you noticed him?"

"Yes, clearly. I mean he had to turn around after he saw me swerve and then had to catch up to me."

"Well then, all he needed to do was look at his own speedometer and he would have had all the evidence he needed. I agree with *Eema*, (Hebrew for Mom), he was lying. You couldn't have been going 80, there's no way."

I thought about it and realized they were probably right. The more I thought about it, the angrier I became.

"That FUCKER!" I yelled. I mean if I was really drunk, why would he need to make up the speeding bit. Being drunk is more than enough to nail me hard…

But the reality is that I am now so insecure about my cognitive abilities that I had originally *believed him* when he told me I was speeding.

Normally I would have simply told him he was wrong. I *had* looked at my speedometer when I swerved and it was 45. I hadn't yet reached the speed at which I routinely engage the cruise control to *make sure* that I wouldn't exceed the speed limit through inattention. Like I said before, I now drive like a frightened Granny.

That's clearly not good enough. It must be the ADD that is causing me to make mistakes like this. I told my wife and son that I would never mess with the Iphone again unless I pulled over first. I've been doing that for a while when I needed to dial a number. Now I'll do it whenever I want to listen to the Ipod part of it as well.

I had a lot of interesting things I was planning on writing about today, and all this *kvetching*, especially after the last chapter, may not play too well in the narrative. Perhaps I'll cut it or put it in a few chapters later in the book, if I ever finish it.

In the meantime, I needed to "blow out" all that happened in writing. It's a useful way to "externalize" bad feelings so they're not just bottled up inside oneself.

The Sanskrit meaning of *Nirvana* is to "blow out," that deep sigh of relief that happens when one realizes that everything is going to be alright.

Having written this, I now feel a little better, though I'm still afraid to get back in a car. I'll have to get passed that feeling. I can't leave all the driving to my wife and Barak still doesn't have his license. I'm out of Valiums too. Maybe I'll smoke some pot and that will help. Maybe I'll try to meditate. Maybe I'll blow my head off... Just kidding!

I'm alone in the house now. It's 11 AM and Suz has to go to the dentist after dropping the kids off in school.

I can't distract myself with the news and blogs online. Hillary's victory in PA is just too awful for me to think about today. I haven't had my first Provogil yet, and I wonder if I should. Maybe the MS "brain fog" is what I need right now rather than clarity.

God, do I HATE feeling sorry for myself. I apologize to whatever audience may end up reading this. Don't worry. I've been through worse and will come through this fine.

I just need a little more time....

14. Covering all the Bases

Passover at my father's house. I was really proud of myself at the first Seder because I managed to stay up till 12! Not easy for me to do, but I took a third Provogil and *something* worked.

The next morning, my father was looking for my son to walk him to synagogue. He *is* 92 after all. I headed him off at the pass.

"Let him sleep, Pop. I'll take you. In fact I'll come to *schull* too."

"Really?" My father could scarcely conceal his surprise. "Great! Let's go then…"

Of course he had every reason to be surprised. I had stopped going with him to synagogue probably five years or so before. It's not that I hated it, exactly. It made me feel incredibly hypocritical.

You see, I'm what the Jewish community would rightly call an *apikoress*. It means apostate, but it means more than that. It means *learned* apostate. It's what they called Spinoza, so it carries with it a proud tradition.

Spinoza is by far my favorite Western philosopher. He reaches for the same truths that Eastern philosophers reach for using rigidly Western methods. His geometric logic makes it hard to understand him sometimes, but it's worth the work! Or so I am told, never actually bothering to try myself and settling instead for second hand treatises *about* his philosophy. One day. Maybe. I doubt it.

Anyway, I actually deserve to be called an *apikoress* rather than an *am oratz* which signifies ignorant violator of the Jewish law.

My father made sure in my upbringing that I would know as much as possible. Learn to *Learn*. In Judaism, learning about the Jewish law is the highest thing one can attain to.

He taught me himself. We went through *chumash and rashi* (Old Testament in Hebrew with its greatest commentator) together at least three times. He also taught me *Mishna* and *Gemara* (Historically later, very complicated and difficult discussions of Jewish Law). He sent me to a Jewish Day School for three years till I threatened to run away from home. He hired private tutors. Some wonderful. Some horrid beyond belief. Thwakford Sqeers with sculcaps.

Anyway, you get the Idea. By the time I was 16 and left home, I knew more about Judaism than everything else combined. I *mean* that. Think about what that says about me….

After youthful abandonment of the tradition, I tried to get back into it with a vengeance. I took my second year off from law school to go study in a yeshiva in Israel. Afterwards I went so far as to do *daf yomi* (daily reading of a complete page of *gemara*) the last two years of Law School.

After that I joined the Israeli Navy and actually managed to get into the officers course. (Not an easy thing to do by any standard). I dropped out later because I couldn't face seven years with the kids I was with, lovely though they were. Remember, I was a Columbia Law School graduate. The intellectual vacuum that seven years as an officer would have meant was more than I could face.

It's fair to ask, "Why didn't you think of this before you joined?" To which I would weakly reply, "Well, you know what they say, *hope springs eternal.*"

The truth was, or at least part of the truth was, that I was trying to emulate my father as best as I could. He fought in the American navy in WWII. I think as a kid I was more proud of him for that than anything else. I have a battle torn 48 star flag hanging next to me in a frame in my office. I had found it, forgotten somewhere up in an attic. There was a yellowed with age note in his handwriting that I had transferred to a silver back, and which underlies it in the frame. The card reads:

October 30, 1944

This is the flag flown by USS Zane in February 1944 during the first days of the assault on Eniwetok Atoll in the Marshall Islands. The Zane and Chandler were the first American warships to go into Eniwetok via deep entrance preceding the cruisers and battleships.

The officer of the Deck at battle stations was

Herman Wouk, then Lt.jg USNR

Anyway, it's obvious that I'm still proud. On the other side of my office I have some nice pictures from my service when I volunteered to go back to my Israeli naval unit during the first gulf war, but that's another story.

Wow! What a ramble. Remember I have MS, OK? I'll read over what I wrote and get to the point soon, I promise.

OK, so I tried and tried to be a good Jew like my Dad. When I got married it was on condition that she agreed to obey the *halacha* (Jewish religious law) with me.

But there came a point when it all came to a crashing end. I told my father about this event in explaining to him why I no longer believed and no longer followed the Jewish tradition.

I was living in Israel with my family in the most incredible house that Suz and I were sure at the time we had "manifested."

In the back, it had a hot tub in a room made of glass brick with plants all around it. Literally heaven. Understand that at the time there couldn't have been more than ten hot tubs in the whole country.

Sitting in the boiling tub with the steam rising around me I experienced a sudden realization unlike anything that had ever hit me before in terms of its consequences. Here is what I suddenly understood:

> *The ENTIRE Jewish religion and all the*
> *religions it spawned were based on*
> *justifying the first act of genocide in*
> *recorded history.*

There's absolutely no argument that can be made against that statement. Believe me, I know. I really know. My father saw to that, remember?

Not even regular genocide, like the Germans did to us or the Turks to the Armenians. No. We were "commanded by god" not only to kill the soldiers, or the men, or the men and women, or the men and women and children. No. God "commanded us" not only to kill the soldiers, the men, the women, the infants, but *even the domestic animals.* All must be put to the sword.

Why?!!!!

"Because they worshiped idols and threw their children to Baal. They were evil and needed to be destroyed." That's the conventional answer.

That's the answer? We killed their babies because *they* killed their babies? What have the animals to do with anything?

"The animals would have been sacrificed to Baal."

Well I'm sure that wasn't *their* idea, and once Israel captured them they were not going to be sacrificed to Baal anyway. Why kill them? Why kill *anybody* just because they worship the "wrong god"?

The justifier in my head continues:

"All right, maybe there were things done then that we wouldn't do today. Don't forget the world was different thousands of years ago. That's an incident and has nothing to do with what Judaism is *based* on."

But you see, that can't hold water with me. I *know* too much.

I remember the first Rashi commentary on the first sentence in Genesis. *"In the beginning god created the heavens and the earth."* Rashi asks, why begin here? Who needs all this stuff? Why not just begin with Leviticus where the Jewish law is laid down?

Rashi's no vagrant, and this is not a rhetorical question. It is based on the assumption that *every word* in our Torah is there for a reason.

Here's Rashi's answer to his question. (paraphrased)

It is because when the nations of the world accuse Israel of being *brigands* by stealing the land from the Canaanites, we can answer that since god created the world, he can give it to who he chooses, and he chose to give this land to the Jews.

You can't get more basic than that. The entire superstructure of Judaism, starting with the Old Testament up till the latest commentators is built on Rashi's answer. The genocide the Jews committed was OK, see, because god created the world and told the Jews to help themselves to Canaan. Oh, and while you're at it, kill everything that is alive in the area you seize.

I call this realization "the flash in the hot tub" and though it may not sound like much to many of my readers, try and understand. I had built my *entire* life around the Jewish tradition and had just figured out that I was supporting the notion of genocide by my continued adherence to it.

These are the kind of realizations that can be brought about by psychedelics. I had never thought of this before because the "reality tunnel" I had been living in wouldn't let the idea through. We were the *good* guys... The ones that everyone has picked on through history... The ones who were *RIGHT!*

When I told this to my Dad, he managed an ironic smile and shrugged. I knew I had broken his heart, but what could I do? That was how I now saw things. I respected him far too much than to lie to him.

Since that time, my Dad has accepted me as I am. He knows I'll never stop loving the tradition I was steeped in. He respected my intellectual honesty and even compared me to Spinoza. Like I mentioned before, he's as close to a renaissance man as I have ever know. He's read Spinoza in the *original.*

We arrived at the *Chabad* synagogue shortly, and I went in to greet the Rabbi there who I really liked. We started *davening* (praying) and it all came back as if I had been there last week. But the 5 years away did make me pay attention to what I was saying in the prayers a bit more than usual.

We got to the *Shema* which is the central prayer that Jews are supposed to say three times a day, that we hang in *mezuzoth* on our doors and that we are supposed to say as our last dying words:

> *Hear O' Israel the Lord is our God, the*
> *Lord is one.*
> *And you should love the lord your God,*
> *with all your heart, with all your soul, and*
> *with all your strength.*

Reading that phrase, I was struck by the fact that it is an example of what Alan Watts used to call a "double bind." A double bind occurs when you are commanded to do something which is acceptable only if it's voluntary. Get it? It can't be done! One cannot be "commanded" to love anything. It has to come from inside.

Think of it this way, if you asked your lover, "Do you love me?" would you be satisfied with the answer, "I'm trying with all my heart…"

So God was commanding us to do the impossible. Why? It didn't make sense?

My old Talmudic training swung into action and I continued to ponder the question through the Torah reading. And then, suddenly I *knew* the answer. I got so excited that I asked the Rabbi if I could deliver a short *drasha* (comment on the Torah) after his. He graciously allowed me to do so.

Up before the congregation, I laid before them the problem I had discovered in the *Shema*. The answer I discovered was that the phrase "God is one" is *not* meant to say he isn't two gods or a thousand for that matter. What it is saying is that God is *everything*. And you, and you, and you, are all apertures through which his light shines, as is everything else that exists!

Looked at that way, the second sentence was no double bind commandment. It was a continuation of the *descriptive* nature of the first sentence. There's no way *not* to love God if you *are* god.

I then told them that I had lost my faith years before, but that if there were any there who felt true faith that they please say a prayer for me, as I had developed incurable multiple sclerosis. There were practically tears in my eyes, and I know I spoke very intensely.

It was time for *Musaf* (extra prayer said on holidays) and I reached in my pocket for a Provogil. Shit! I had forgotten them at home and was going to need one soon. I'd never make the walk home without one.

I explained to my Dad, and he waved me off. On my way out, hands reached out to shake mine, *yasher coach's* (well done!) from all sides. As I passed through the women's section on the way out, one thanked me for what I had said. "Wow! Even the women heard me." I thought.

I stumble bummed my way home. The MS is really beginning to take a toll on my balance. Ten minutes later, my Dad showed up.

"Pop! What are you doing home so soon? They can't have finished yet..."
"Just wanted to be sure you made it. I have to daven *Musaph* now..."

The next day, I stayed home. My Dad was accompanied home by one of the Rabbi's sons. Meeting me in the hallway he eagerly pumped my hand.

"I want you to know that what you did yesterday was a real *Kiddush Hashem!*" (Sanctification of the Lord). That's about as high a compliment that a religious Jew can give. I told him not to exaggerate, but he was insistent.

Is that what I am?

Maybe in some ways we *all* are.

This was just my Andy Warhol's 15 minutes.

I wonder how many other self proclaimed *apikoresses* have been told they are a *Kiddush Hashem*?

I know one thing though…

If Spinoza was alive today, both my father and I would stand in line to tell him he was a *Kiddush Hashem* with all our hearts.

15. The Buddha Nature

Truthfully, I have no business writing this chapter. I'm certainly no Buddhist scholar, and I don't kid myself into thinking there's any more "truth" to this than anything else I write. It is simply my personal experience here. When you come right down to it, what else can you *really* trust?

I was sitting in Bob's back garden, a lovely little place with climbing flower vines and a remarkable tree that had these fuzzy bright red flowers. I was trying to explain to him the transformation I had gone through in the last few weeks.

"When I first was diagnosed with MS, I just chalked it up as the 'balancing event' in an otherwise perfect life." The notion that "balance" must exist in each organism's existence is silly to the point of ridiculousness. Any "balance" that exists, exists on a universal level. One that we are unable to access on a normal basis, only when in the grips of ecstasy.

But we can't help ourselves. No matter how much our intellect tells us it's silly, for some reason we hang on to many superstitions. In the backs of our heads, of course. No "reasonable" person would ever believe such stupid stuff. Right?

"Now I realize that it may just have been the one thing that could jolt me out of the bad pattern I was in before. I would never have changed without the MS." As Lao Tzu says, inside every curse is nestled a blessing, and I really felt I had found it.

"You know Bob, I'm really not afraid of death anymore. I could be run over tomorrow. What difference would that make to me? Nothing at all…"

Bob peered at me from across the table where he was rolling a joint. "I can see that you mean that," he said. "You've made some good progress. You have a *very* long way to go."

"Maybe," I answered, "But I just wanted to tell you how good it feels…. Blow it out, you know. Nirvana…"

"Leave Nirvana out of this," Bob said, "You've got to work on your addictive behaviors…."

"Here he goes again…." I thought to myself. More lectures on the Winstons. It's not that I disagree with anything he says; it's just that I'm unwilling to give up this last crutch until at least the first ayahuasca session. I see no advantage in needless suffering at this point. It would only distract me from what I was trying to do.

I started to answer him when he held up his hand to stop me. "I just want you to know that whatever you say to me will make no difference. I will regard it as an addict's rationalization."

Ouch! "Alright, then I won't waste our time. What's your point?"

"All these addictive behaviors have a motive behind them. A reason they are there. They don't 'just happen'." He lit the joint and passed it over. "Do you think it's the same reason you think you have MS?"

I instantly knew it wasn't. It was much deeper. It somehow struck to the core of my perception of "being" in itself. And then I suddenly knew the answer…

"No. Not at all. It's more the bottom line of human existence, if you will. Here we are, but we're all going to die no matter what we do… You know," I chuckled as I realized what I was saying. "The problems the Buddha was concerned with."

Bob peered at me intensely. He had to know I was telling him the truth as I had just discovered it. He *saw* me do it....

"You know, I called an MD friend of mine who's also a Shaman and I spoke to him about your case. That I wasn't sure if you were prepared enough."

"What'd he say?" I asked, very interested.

"He said I should tell you that whatever pain you avoid now through your habits, you will pay for in your ayahuasca experience. The experience 'cleanses" you of all the shit... The more shit you have, the harder it's going to be..."

"You mean it's going to hurt more or terrify more?" I asked.

He nodded gravely.

"Bring it on..." I answered truthfully. I really am not afraid. Well, maybe a little, but not enough to give up the cigs yet. No way...

But I really do feel like I've broken through some level or other. Last night, I half kiddingly told my wife that I finally had an ambition.

"What... to write your book?" She asked.

"No," I answered. "I want to be a Buddha..."

I told Bob this story and he laughed.

"I'll be right back." I said and went off for an MS piss.

While waiting for the goddamned "hesitation" to end, I thought about the effect my words may have had on Bob.

On returning to our table I immediately said to him (so I wouldn't forget), "Listen, I don't want you to have any misapprehensions about me because of my saying I want to be a Buddha. The point is that I'm not really seeking Nirvana or anything else for that matter. I want to have the "effect" of a Buddha on all those around me. The way Jack

Kornfield makes me feel when I hear him speak. Calm, and somehow 'knowing' that everything's OK."

"Anyhow, that's really what I'm after. To develop a 'Buddha nature' rather than "being" a *pratyeka* (private) Buddha sitting off by myself in a corner somewhere."

Lao Tzu says "An integral being benefits all things, yet people are scarcely aware of his existence."

This is going to be quite a challenge, I would say. To develop a calming Buddha nature while suffering from Progressive Relapsing MS. I wonder if it's been done before? Maybe I'll be the first?

Maybe not…

Stay tuned for the next episode of: *Will I be a Buddha or a "drool bucket"?*

16. Nightmare Time

These are the times that try men's souls. I'm sure I heard that somewhere… Just kidding!

So this is how bad it's getting. Sorry if it brings you down, you need to know to understand the rest of this book if I finish it.

Just got back from UCSF with my son Barak. Dr. Goodin wasn't there so I got to see Dr. Crabtree. (Terrible name, but one sharp woman…) She agreed that it was most likely that the self diagnoses I had made of suffering from PRMS (Progressive Relapsing Multiple Sclerosis) was correct. Here's why:

1. PRMS tends to hit older males
2. PRMS tends to hit those with spinal compression (Did I mention that mine was compressed to 1/3 of its normal size?)
3. PRMS is characterized by early depression onset
4. PRMS is characterized by early cognitive dysfunction (Before many lesions appear.)
5. My cognitive dysfunction continues to deteriorate absent a relapse.
6. My balance continues to deteriorate absent a relapse.

I'm sure there's more I'm forgetting, but the above is enough. To give you an idea of how bad it's getting:

After we got home, I went to turn on the computer, and noticed that my computer glasses were missing. I remembered that I had left them hung on a specific curtain in the RV. Proud of having remembered this, I got up and walked the 40 feet or so to the RV. By the time I got there I had forgotten why I had gone. What was I looking for? I couldn't remember.

No problem… Happens all the time. I just retraced my steps, sat down in front of the computer and was reminded that I couldn't view the screen without my glasses. Right! My glasses! I got up and walked back to the RV. By the time I got there I had forgotten why I had gone. What was I looking for? I couldn't remember.

"This is ridiculous!" I thought to myself. "I should probably look in the driver's seat. Maybe I'll see it…" And damned if I didn't! There they were… The Iphone headphones I had forgotten to bring them in… Ha! Got them….! I proudly returned to the office bearing my prize to sit in front of a fuzzy screen…

"Shit! My glasses!" I realized in horror what had just happened. "Not this time!" I said to myself. This time, every third step I said the word "glasses" out loud. When I got to the RV, I went straight up to the curtain and retrieved my glasses. I felt a little silly doing it, speaking out loud like that, but I really didn't want to forget them *three* times in a row.

My "drunken sailor" routine continues to get worse. Bob made me switch to running shoes instead of my comfortable but supportless Uggs. Barak said my walking looked better as a result, and I was gratified to hear that. I still almost fell a few times today for no apparent reason.

At least I can still drive as long as *all* I do is drive. I have a new rule since being pulled over by that cop. From now on if I want to do *anything* other than drive I pull over first. That includes adjusting the radio, Iphone, whatever that requires me to take my eyes off the road for more than a fraction of a second. I'll still look quickly down to check my speed, but that's it.

Anyhow, this is how it is. I called my father, desperate for advice. What should I do? Keep on keeping on and hope nothing happens? Stop driving altogether and treat myself like an invalid?

His advice was to start writing and sticking to a daily schedule, checking off items as you complete them. He said he'd been doing that for years and it really helped him. Don't forget, he's 93 and still writing books!

I asked my wife if she would help me do this and she said "Of course I will…"

No surprise there. She's been after me for years to make lists and follow them. I'm not really sure why I have resisted so much until now. I guess it kind of makes me feel like a prisoner. But I have to remember that I'm just being a prisoner to myself at this point. That's not even possible, is it?

The last question was whether I was suffering from subcortical dementia. Not all PRMS sufferers get it, though some do. I asked the doctor how one found out and she told me there was a battery of unpleasant tests one needed to take. I told her to schedule them for me and hope to find out a date next week.

After all this, I'm supposed to find equanimity. I'm working at it. There's no doubt that the writing helps. I guess putting pain on the page makes you feel better because it's shared. That makes no sense, I know, but we're talking human neurosis here!

So, to who ever ends up reading this. Thank you for sharing my pain. I feel better already.

17. Yin Yang, Novelty/Habit, and Quality

So it's been a few days since I wrote that last semi-panicked chapter. I'm fine now, *really* fine. Had an amazing day today full of discovery and goodness. Working on developing my Buddha nature has already begun to pay back in such happiness and equanimity that I am actually considering abandoning my quest for a cure via the shamanic ayahuasca and instead focus on trying to cure myself or at least find serenity in Buddhism.

But that's not what this chapter's about. It's just an update on my condition.

Now to get to the meat….

Most people, including westerners are familiar with the Chinese concept of Yin Yang. The notion is that all of reality can be broken into two categories that each depends on the other for their own existence, and that together form *what is*.

The symbol of the white/black "S" shape drawn through a circle creating two fish shaped figures white and black is probably even more well know.

The origin of the terms is the Chinese words for the two sides of a mountain. The sunny side and the shady side. It is important to understand that there is *no way* that a mountain can exist without both sides. That is why those words were chosen to represent two *opposites*, that each must exist for the other to exist.

Sounds kind of nutty said that way, but this is where illustrations help.

Can there be up without down?

Can there be long without short?

Can there be wide without narrow?

Can there be succinctness without long-windedness? Heh!

Get the idea?

It's like two poles of a magnet. You can't have a plus without a minus. There's no way you can cut off one from the other. You just end up with two smaller magnets, each with two poles.

The Chinese believe that all of reality consists of these "opposites" that each rely on the other to exist. That's the basic concept of Yin Yang. The I Ching, which came later, consists of 64 "hexagrams" of Yin Yang organizations. These 64 are supposed to be the only ways that reality can be arranged.

The Chinese would say that perfect health cannot exist without illness/death. Each relies on the other to exist. Because of that, they can be viewed as *ONE* even though they are opposites.

The circle is the one, and death and life are the two halves of the one that depend on each other to exist.

At least a portion, if not the greatest portion of my current equanimity can be attributed to my understanding and acceptance of the Yin Yang model as the best model for reality that humans have managed to concoct. Death is no longer the "threat" I used to feel it was. That removes a great deal of anxiety *instantaneously*.

I know it sounds silly to say that any metaphysical conception can do us any good, but I can simply report how it affected me.

There is a Western version of essentially the same idea. Robert Pirsig's *Metaphysics of Quality* breaks reality down into two opposites that need each other. Static Quality and Dynamic Quality. Yin and Yang.

Zen and the Art of Motorcycle Maintenance was where Pirsig introduced the idea, and *Lila* was the book in which he brought it to fruition. Before I studied much Eastern religion, I was a Pirsig fanatic. I must have read or listened to those books a dozen times. He was trying to change the way we view reality, from object as being primary to relationship as being primary.

That's a mouthful, I know... Sorry. Let's see how I do in explaining this mouthful...

The classic Western "common sense" comes down to us from Sir Isaac Newton. That common sense tells us that the universe is made up of objects that may or may not develop relationships. But the objects exist regardless of whether there are any relationships developed.

Pirsig chose the word "quality" to describe the relationship between two objects. But under Pirsig's Metaphysics, the relationship is what creates the objects. That's what I meant above when using the term "primary." Which comes first?

It makes no sense to the Western mind to view relationship as primary. That's a real disability we all suffer from because our own science has proven to us over and over that relationship *is* primary.

Once again, let's play with examples.

Imagine an infinite, empty universe that contains only one object. Can that object move?

Imagine the same only with two objects passing each other. Which one is moving? Is either still?
The point I'm making here, is that it is relationship and relationship alone that "creates" motion.

Get it?

Moving right along here, Einstein's Special Relativity teaches that it is the relationship between the objects that determines how each will experience the other.

Muons are extremely short lived particles that are created when gamma rays hit our atmosphere. They are *so* short lived that there's no way any should make it to ground level before decaying even given their near light speed.

And yet Muons make it down all the time. What?! Not possible!

Yes, possible. The relationship between the muon and the earth which is near light speed slows the muon's experience of time to one seventh our experience of time on earth. So the muon survives seven times longer than it should in our reality because in *its* reality it decays as quickly as it *should* decay in our reality.

That is considered the hardest physical proof we have of the Special Theory of Relativity. You have to admit, it's a pretty damn good proof. But once again, it is divorced from Western common sense because it places primacy on relationship over objects.

Sorry, we're back to quantum physics again…

The primacy of relationship over object is everywhere you look in the quantum dimension. The math *always* works. It's the most verified theory in the history of physics. The problems only emerge when you try to describe what happens in language rather than math. The result is hopeless paradoxes in all directions, but ONLY if one insists on the primacy of object over relationship. (Our "common sense.")

Let's go out in the garden…

Which came first, the flower or the bee?

Which side holds up the other side on that sawhorse?

What makes the shoreline of the pond?

Clearly it's the relationships in the above examples that are primary. We know that, but it makes us "feel funny" to think that way so we avoid it.

Einstein had a "beginner's mind" as Gary Zukov points out in *The Dancing Wu-Li Masters*. That's what made it possible for him to come up with Special Relativity. All he did was change the biggest paradox of his time, the constant speed of light, into a postulate from which he redrew reality according to the *relationships* between objects.

Bottom line, our "common sense" is wrong. And not just down on the quantum level. Pretty much everywhere you look.

I *know* better, but it's still my common sense. I don't know how to change that. Maybe if I was a real physicist and could move in their world of math I could understand better, even if I couldn't put it into words. Maybe.

To close this circle, I'd like to bring up Terence McKenna's *Time Wave*, based on his *Novelty Theory*.

Novelty theory has a few basic tenets:
- That the universe is a living system with a teleological attractor at the end of time that drives the increase and conservation of complexity in material forms.
- That novelty and complexity increase over time, despite repeated set-backs.
- That the human brain represents the pinnacle of complex organization in the known universe to date.
- That fluctuations in novelty over time are self-similar at different scales. Thus the rise and fall of the Roman Empire might be resonant with the life of a family within a single generation, or with an individual's day at work.
- That as the complexity and sophistication of human thought and culture increase, universal novelty approaches a Koch curve of infinite exponential growth.
- That in the time immediately prior to, and during this omega point of infinite novelty, anything and everything conceivable to the human imagination will occur simultaneously.
- That the date of this historical endpoint is December 21, 2012, the end of the long count of the Mayan calendar. (Although many interpretations of the "end" of the Mayan calendar exist, partly due to abbreviations made by the Maya when referring to the date, McKenna used the solstice date in 2012, a common

interpretation of the calendar among New Age writers, although this date corresponds to such an abbreviation rather than the full date. See Mayan calendar for more information on this controversy.) Originally McKenna had chosen the end of the calendar by looking for a very novel event in recent history, and using this as the beginning of the final 67.29 year cycle; the event he chose was the atomic bombing of Hiroshima, which gave an end-date in mid-November of 2012, but when he discovered the proximity of this date to the end of the current 13-baktun cycle of the Maya calendar, he adjusted the end date to match this point in the calendar.[1][2]

This *End of History* was to be the final manifestation of The Eschaton, which McKenna characterized as a sort of strange attractor towards which the evolution of the universe developed. – Wikipepia

As nutty as all this sounds, it's very closely related to Yin/Yang. Novelty and Habit are almost synonyms for Yang and Yin. Not only that, The timewave itself is a combination of numerology and mathematics. It is formed out of McKenna's interpretation and analysis of numerical patterns in the King Wen sequence of the I Ching (the ancient Chinese *Book of Changes*), which we know represent all the possible combinations of Yin/Yang.

The biggest change from our "common sense" in McKenna's *Time Wave* is that progress is not the result of past achievements so much as it is being pulled forward by some source *ahead* of us in time. This is not as absurd to modern physics as it is to common sense. The easiest way to work with anti-particles is to treat them as particles moving backward in time. That doesn't *prove* they move backward in time, but given time's altered effects in the quantum level, it wouldn't necessarily be impossible.

The notion is that what causes time to flow forward is the second law of thermodynamics. That law states that in a closed system disorder will increase over time. That disorder increase is what makes time irreversible on the macro level. On the quantum level however, the second law doesn't apply. Thus there is no "arrow of time" on that level.

All these non-Western metaphysical outlooks would allow me to cure this MS, I think. It's hard for me to put my finger on what it is about each one that gives me hope, but the overall effect is to show me once again that our "common sense" *ain't necessarily so...*

18. Sauren to New Heights

Sitting in Beckman's Cafe with Bob, is a man in his thirties who looks straight as an arrow. Bob introduces him to me as Bill, and explains that he is the son of the College professor who had had her liver lesion shrunk by an ayahuasca cure.

Bill tells me the story of how his Mom, having nothing to lose, had agreed to try the Amazonian cure at his urging after her doctors threw up their hands.

"She said that on her plane trip, before landing, she glanced out over the jungle and felt an overwhelming power emanating from below."

We spoke about what Bob and I were planning, and whether or not it was worth trying the cure here surrounded by my redwood trees, or going to the jungle for the "real thing." He told me that it is indeed outrageously hot there and that there is no air conditioning.

"What about electricity? Do they have that?" I asked.

It turns out they did, and we discussed the possibility of buying a window air conditioner in Lima and bringing it out to the jungle with us so I would have some escape from the heat between sessions.

It turned out that Bill's 17 year old nephew is suffering from Juvenile Diabetes so badly that it has essentially wiped out his life. Bill is trying to convince him to go down to the Amazon for a cure. He is a super rationalist and thinks it's all crap. I would hope that Bill's mom's experience would convince him to at least give it a try.

Bill mentions that he might be interested in making a documentary film about this.

I take a long moment to consider this. Would the presence of a documentary crew asking questions and filming help or hinder what I was trying to do here? Is it really that different than me writing about it? It is and it isn't, of course. Just like everything else, it depends how you look at it. But it occurs to me that if I get others involved in the process, it is likely to help encourage me to proceed with it where I might otherwise get cold feet.

"I think it could make an amazing documentary." I said. "Especially if you can convince your nephew to come and track us both through the attempted healing."

Bob had to leave for an appointment, so Bill and I retired to sit at an outdoor table where we could smoke while we drank our coffee.

He and I were talking about MS and the various possibilities being offered by Western science to battle it.

"Alkalinity!" A voice called from a table across from us. "You have to change your diet and make it alkaline. It saved my life!"

I looked over to the source of the voice and saw a handsome, thin, man about my age or a little less. His skin was darker than standard white and his hair was jet black. He was leaning back in his chair sipping his coffee from a paper cup.

"Come join us," I called out to him, and he slid into the third seat at our table.

"Now tell me about what saved your life? What happened?"

For five minutes I sat there and listened to his particular story of woe. Lymphoma metastasized all over the place. The doctors said he had at most six months. That was nine months ago.

"If you think I'm skinny now, you should have seen me," he grinned. "I was twenty pounds lighter…"

OK, I thought to myself, which would have made you look like an Auschwitz survivor at the time. I asked him about the Alkalinity diet.

"Just look it up on the internet, it's everywhere…"

He then launched into a stunning disposition on the subject which I couldn't reproduce here even if I wanted to. But what intrigued me much more than the "cure" was the man talking. The way he spoke, the honesty which poured out, the incredible intensity that he put behind every word.

We just kept talking. He would stop and I would start. Before I would finish, he'd jump to the end of what I was going to say and add on his view. I found myself doing the same with him.

I am now 54 years old, and I can say with absolute conviction that I have never met anyone in my life with a mind as close to mine as this strange, sick man.

His name was Sauren Crow. He was not only as smart and quick witted; he was deeply knowledgeable in both areas I was familiar with as well as others like music and art with which I am less conversant. When he started talking about quantum physics intelligently, I knew I had found something very special in my life. A new friend!

"Hey, I saw you came on a bike. If you live near here we could go to your place and smoke a bowl, my treat…"

And we were off. Him on his bike and me trailing him in the car. We arrived at his place and he opened the garage with a remote.

There was a couch on one wall and I could see a loft in the back with a bed on it.

"You live here? In the garage? How much do they charge you for this?"

"Six hundred dollars," he said. "It's not too bad, it's just the goddamned cold…"

Not too bad? A freezing garage with a cement floor for $600? This amazing man? What the hell?!!!! None of this made any sense. He was a goddamned indigent? Lived from dollar to dollar, from day to day?

We sat, side by side on the couch doing bowl after bowl, barely stopping talking as we puffed. Hours went by and we just kept going at it. Both into Buddhism, Taoism, scuba diving, and any drug we could get our hands on. We started talking about art and he pulled out a ream of slides in plastic jackets filled with pictures of gigantic, beautiful modern art displays he had had commissioned in New Mexico.

"Hey, this would be amazing for Burning Man! We should submit these slides with an application. They might give you a grant!"

Then we started telling each other about our backgrounds. Me, with Columbia Law, Israel Navy, film production, dropping out, internet business.

Him: father a full blooded Sioux asshole alcoholic, studied math and physics at Berkley, got into play directing, got addicted to heroin and ended up living on the streets in downtown LA. As one of the only white derelicts in the area, most of the blacks stayed away, figuring he was either crazy or had a gun.

One day a huge black guy tried to start up with him. Did I tell you he was a Jeet Kundo expert? Anyway, after disassembling this huge villain he acquired the nickname downtown as "White Lion." He broke into a perfect female black dialogue, "You know who you messin with? That there's the White Lion!" He laughed with complete pleasure, "You shoulda seen how they backed away!" He was standing and waving his arms around as he spoke. The same way I always do.

Not to be outdone, I had to tell him the story of how I had dropped acid during reserve duty in Israel while having rockets drop on all sides of the base. He was rolling with laughter. "Shit... Wars! Do they ever suck!!"

Turns out he had been assigned on some kind of UN mission during the Bosnia wars. He began relating some hilarious bureaucratic stories and then started in on some horrible stuff.

"I don't want to hear it." I held up my hand. "I'm sorry; I just can't take listening to that kind of stuff. I won't go to a sad movie. I won't even listen to a sad song. I've been depressed, and don't want to go back there…"

"You're absolutely right!" He said. "Fuck that shit. We have only goodness here…"

And I knew he was right.

"Look at this tattoo." He said holding out his hand. On the back was the figure of some sort of multi pointed arrow. "That's what you get after the vision quest."

He told me how at one point his Sioux heritage got a hold on his mind and nothing would do but to pass the vision quest. Four days on the top of the mountain, no food, no water. By the third day, the hallucinations begin. By the fourth you are completely at one with the universe and know that you are a part of the whole.

"Cool…" I said. "But what did you get out of it besides the truism that I instantly understood the minute you told me?"

He looked down and thought hard for a minute. "Nothing, I guess…" He shrugged. We both rolled in laughter for the uncountable time.

Suddenly he doubled over and ran out the garage door and began walking in a circle in the middle of the street.

"Hey, you OK?" I shouted. He lifted his arm and waved to signal that he heard, but he could not speak.

"Is it the pain?" I yelled. He nodded in assent. Well maybe his diet had improved things for him, but that pain showed he still had the cancer. What can I do to help him? And then I felt the little dropper bottle in the pocket of my sweatshirt. I had gotten some THC tincture from a

Medical Marijuana dispensary the day before. It was the best thing I knew of for pain.

I called him over and made him take a dropper. He stood as rigid as bronze, and I watched him turn back into flesh and blood in about 30 seconds. "Take another…" I told him, and he quickly complied.

"Finger of God, man… Thank you, thank you…"

"Keep the bottle." I said. "You need it a lot right now, and I'm pain free at the moment… Buddha nature!"

After a few minutes we resumed our animated conversation. I told him of my plans to try and "cure" this PRMS through ayahuasca. He was all for it and offered to help me get to the jungle. Help me? He needed the cure a LOT more than I did.

He told me how nine years ago he had decided to go transsexual and had started on hormone treatments. He never finished the job though, and had now given up on it. "Who wants an old broad anyway," he laughed. "I'm 59…"

"You bastard!" I shouted, you look younger than me! He did too, though that may say more about me than it does about him.

"This is all that's left from that effort." He lifted his shirt. "Not much, but a little…"

"Jezuz fucking Christ who the hell ARE you?" I shouted. "White lion with tits!"

He *really* liked that one and we rolled around in mutual merriment again. This was my kind of man. Knows as much as possible. Takes nothing too seriously. *Knows* he's really clueless…

I had to go get Zohar from school. Exchanging numbers, he promised to call and remind me to come back at 4:30 so we could continue our fun. I'd been doing the *Memento* bit lately, and was afraid I would forget.

In the end, he couldn't call because his phone had run out of minutes. It took me half an hour to find his house as I had completely forgotten how I had gotten there. When I finally found it at around 5 PM, nobody answered at his garage door.

Driving home, I wondered if I had imagined the whole thing. I knew that couldn't be, though. MS or no MS. But it was incredibly strange, nonetheless. It was as though I had ordered the perfect friend to be designed and built by God and delivered to me via Federal Express. It had NEVER happened to me before. Nothing even close. I have never needed it so much before either. Rule of 23s? This was no 23. This was a unique occurrence in my life.

In legend, Bodhisattvas tend to show up in all sorts of disguises, most of them lowly… Hookers, tramps and the like.

"What the fuck is going on here?" I wondered to myself, "The first thing he tried to do was help me heal. And then he turns out to be everything I want. Coincidence? Must be. What else could it be?" I kept wondering as I watched a line of pelicans fly in formation West over the Pacific into the setting sun.

19. Hyperbaric Foot Shitting

So here I was sitting in an Ionic Foot bath while Sauren was riding the hyperbaric chamber. I know, I know, it sounds nutty, but it's alternative medicine par excellence as advised to me by none other than my ally Sauren Crow. If he had told me to *flap my arms and go to the moon* I probably would have tried.

Instead I was doing my best to ensure that *both* of us survived by following his advice. That was the deal I made with him. I'd follow his advice and he'd follow mine. I have it in mind to take him with me for the ayahuasca cure. The only problem is the money. But maybe I can raise it rather than front it myself.

Glancing down I notice the once pure water looks like baby diarrhea. "What the hell *is* this shit?!" I yelled.

Denis laughed and came over from her desk, "It's you. Impurities."

"All that filth came out of my feet?" It was really hard to believe. But Denis was a friend. I knew this was no con, but knew not what to make of it. "That's really disgusting…."

"How could my feet have shit?" I thought to myself. "What craziness is this? I mean, how could they?"

Just one more mystery to throw on the pile, as far as I'm concerned at this point. "So my feet shit. Ok, what's next?"

What was next was a ride in the claustrophobia inducing hyperbaric chamber. But I was ready for it and gobbled a valium 20 minutes prior.

No sweat. I started calling people from inside the chamber on my back, oxygen mask on my mouth. A little muffled, sure, but they could understand me. It was fun weirding them out telling them where I was calling from.

So now I was on *three* tracks. Western medicine (still waiting for my Tysabri), Shamonic (if I ever find a Shaman here or in Peru) and now, drum roll, *alternative medicine.*

God help me, I'm not sure which seems the silliest to me at this point. I might as well try them all as long as they don't conflict. If there is a conflict, I'll deal with it then.

The synchronicities between me and Sauren had continued with a vengeance. Little things. Like him saying that after enlightenment all that was left to do was laundry.

"Where did you hear that?" I challenged him. In my pocket my Iphone was tuned to a lecture series entitled "*After the Ecstasy, the Laundry*" by Jack Kornfeld.

"I dunno, my head. I made it up…"

I showed him my IPhone tuned to its iPod spot.

As he read it his breath whistled "Damn…."

He had never even heard of Jack Kornfeld…

Believe it or not, that was a SMALL one. I'd rather not talk any more about the others; just take my word that I experienced them almost everywhere I looked.

I guess the best way to play this is to pretend that we are two buddies who happened to meet each other at a time of great need for both of us. What's the big deal, right? I'm sure it happens every Tuesday and Thursday to somebody somewhere. Just lucky, that's all. Nothing new there either.

Just lucky…

20. Cognitive Dissonance

Cognitive Dissonance:

"Dissonance" is a state of psychological discomfort that results from a conflict between a currently held belief and evidence that an opposing belief may be true. Beliefs can encompass ideas, attitudes, and opinions held by an individual and are expressed through thoughts and behaviors.

A critical component of cognitive dissonance theory is that the contradictory evidence that is presented to an individual must be credible evidence. Otherwise there would be no need for the individual to struggle with these competing beliefs. Once dissonance occurs, individuals are highly motivated to resolve this struggle.

There are two general categories of resolutions, the individual can either discard the original belief or disregard the contradictory evidence.

Encyclopedia of Educational Technology

If you couldn't tell from my writing, that was happening to me *big time* last week. It got to the point that I wrote the chapter heading *Cognitive*

Dissonance and I froze. Couldn't write another word. I didn't know what to write. I didn't know what I thought.

It's four days later now, and I'm fine again, thank you. Actually, thank you to my wife and friend Sherrie who helped talk me down from the heights of that spooky business I had gotten sidetracked onto with Sauren.

Spooky it was, (cue in Theremin music) though it's completely behind me now, I think. This was the sort of non-rational point of view I was hoping to attain with the *help* of the ayahuasca, not in *real life* beforehand…

What brought me back solidly to consensus reality was my own realization that if something spooky was *indeed* happening, how could I be sure that it was to my benefit and not an "evil spirit" sent to put me off the true path? I couldn't be sure at all…

That being the case, all the "signals" that I picked up might have been there to help or to hurt me, with no possible way of figuring out which.

In contrast, *toss the spookiness* and all's well. I can still help Sauren, and he me, *without* my having to attach any mystical character to the relationship.

By the end of the last chapter I knew that I had to get out of the weirdness. I wrote that I would "pretend" it was an ordinary friendship. Remember? "Just lucky…"

But now I don't feel like I'm pretending. Most of the synchronicities were Wilson's rule of 23s. The others were truly unusual, but the unusual happens every day. Especially in Santa Cruz, as my wife pointed out. I have managed to find mundane explanations for almost every "fantastic" event that ever happened to me.

I am keenly aware of the "reality building" I do every day.

Forget about finding the "true" reality.

It doesn't exist… It's a made up concept in our minds. (Thanks, Plato…)

Find the reality that *works* best for you. (Thanks, William James…)

What I hope will work for me is the ayahuasca convincing me I am cured. Shouldn't be too hard, I now realize. Just meeting a cool new friend was enough to send me to the moon, rationally speaking, of course.

Bob believes ayahuasca actually cures from its own properties rather than via the placebo effect. He may well be right, at least as far as cancer is concerned. There is so little information about ayahuasca vs. MS that I have to stick with my placebo approach.

The point is that it will cease to be a placebo as far as I am concerned when the drug experience convinces me otherwise. If you thought I sounded nutty the last couple of chapters, well…

"You ain't seen nuttin yet!"

21. Beginner's Mind

Shunrio Suzuki, the great Zen master who first introduced Zen to the West is quoted as saying, "Achieving enlightenment is not difficult. What is difficult is maintaining a beginner's mind."

Most Westerners, when they hear this for the first time have no idea what he means. It sounds ridiculous. Our society values and admires our "experts." The whole point in being a "beginner" is to later become and expert, right? Why hold on to the ignorance of the beginners mind?

But Suzuki is not talking about our *knowledge* when he says "beginner's mind." He's talking about the way we *relate* to that knowledge. Do we use the information, or does the information narrow our scope of inquiry?

The simple way Suzuki put it was, *"In the beginners mind there are many possibilities. In the expert's, there are few."*

Gary Zukov in *The Dancing Wu-Li Masters* uses Einstein as a classic example of the beginner's mind. A beginner sees things the way they *are*, not the way they *must be*. Scientists at the turn of the century knew that the luminiferous aether *must* be. They knew light was a wave and that waves needed to travel in *something*. Thus, there *MUST* be ether for it to travel in.

Einstein saw what *was*. The speed of light was proven to be constant regardless of the motion of the viewer by the Michaelson Morley experiment. All Einstein did was raise this fact's status from paradox to postulate and *voilla* the Special Theory of Relativity was born.

Now that the speed of light was no paradox, Einstein gave us other paradoxes that we have lived with since. In Special Relativity, the *Twins Paradox* allows for one twin to grow older on earth during a short, but very fast trip for her twin sister.

Of course his greatest paradox was his discovery and acceptance of what *was* rather than what *must be* when he proved that light is a particle as well as a wave. This was what won Einstein the Nobel Prize, and underlies all the "weirdness" associated with quantum physics.

In many ways, I guess that's what this book is an attempt to do. To recapture the beginners mind in terms of my own attitudes and allow the Shamanistic cure to do its thing.

Despite being a hardened rationalist.

Despite being an expert and "knowing" better.

I like to think and hope that my recent flirtation with delusion was more caused by my attempt to maintain a "beginner's mind" than by the beginnings of dementia or a slide into schizophrenia.

In my support, I can point to the fact that from the beginning I saw the delusions as "potential" delusions. Nevertheless, I was unwilling to dismiss them as delusions from the beginning. I took my time to think them through and analyze them with an open mind first.

Well, a somewhat open mind, anyway. An open mind combined with my aforementioned nemesis, "hope springing eternal." That's not the same as an open mind of course. That's wish fulfillment with a nice euphemism attached.

In my current condition, I don't think it's possible to eliminate wish fulfillment entirely. I do *so* desperately want to cure this thing that I'm willing to suspend disbelief in every direction.

Anyway, it occurred to me that perhaps this is one of the ways ayahuasca works its magic on some people. Through its hallucinogenic images, it *forces* the patient into adopting the "beginner's mind."

They say that *"seeing is believing,"* and while I consider that an overstatement, especially for experienced psychedelic users, the ayahuasca visions are supposed to be unparalleled in their believability.

They most definitely cause "cognitive dissonance" for anyone who experiences them. Remember from the previous chapter, there are two ways people can deal with cognitive dissonance. The individual can either discard the original belief or disregard the contradictory evidence.

In my case, my original belief is that of Rationalism. Spooks and spirits, superstitions, gods and all the other "supernatural" stuff don't fit and get tossed. The contradictory evidence will be the strength of the ayahuasca visions. If they are strong enough, hopefully I'll "discard the original belief" (Rationalism) long enough for the placebo effect to engage and really cure me.

Once cured, I can then slowly work myself back into my original beliefs if I so desire. Actually, it will probably happen even if I don't desire it. Living in Western society makes it next to impossible for me to hold onto any belief system *other* than Rationalism.

At the moment, I'm deep into Rationalism again. I regard this whole ayahuasca attempt as an act of desperation, (which it undoubtedly is) with little chance of success. Like Suzuki says, in the expert's mind there are few possibilities.

I am counting on the ayahuasca to *make me a beginner* again…

21. Back to Square One?

It's now June 10th, and I am finally able to write the next chapter. About a week ago, I met with Bob after my return from Palm Springs. We had a few bowls at his place and then walked to have lunch at the local health food store a few blocks away.

I told Bob that I was now following 4 tracks when it came to my illness: Western medicine, alternative medicine, Buddhism, and the shamanic cure in Peru. I thought it was a fine meeting. Clearly, Bob thought otherwise.

Four days ago I received the following email from him.

> *Dear Joe,*
>
> *It was good to see you yesterday, but I have to say I am very sorry you've relapsed into smoking cigarettes. I see this as symptomatic of a larger problem.*
>
> *As I have said before, in spite of the things you say, it seems to me that you do not truly or sincerely intend to make yourself healthy. A person who knowingly inhales poisonous gas into their lungs while giving money to the world's most wretched*

*and evil people so they get more children
addicted to their deadly drug, is not on a
path of health or sanity.*

*They are, instead mired and confused in a
profoundly dysfunctional ego. You are
making a great effort to rationalize all
this, as if you were a rationalist.*

*But you are not a rationalist Joe. You are
a rationalizer who makes elaborate
excuses and tries to talk themselves and
others into believing what you dearly wish
was true, but in my frame of reference, is
not.*

*I am not sure what to do. While I think
ayahuasca is, or could be useful for
helping someone deal with their
addictions and their rationalizations, it is
not the trip I signed on for.*

*I do think that ayahuasca can help your
condition if used in a certain way that I
have spent many hours, days and weeks,
trying to convey to you. If or when you
decided to embark on such a healing
journey, let me know.*

With love,

Bob

The email hit me like a sledge hammer. What was I going to do now?

There were three possibilities that I could see. One, I could stop
smoking again and make Bob willing to go with me again. Two, I
could arrange to go on my own. At this point I have enough contacts to

make the trip without him. Finally, I could forget about Peru and instead volunteer to work full time to elect Obama.

I have chosen the final option.

At the risk of being a "rationalizer," I'll try to explain my thinking again.

In the last chapter I mentioned that looked at the right way, MS could be seen as the best thing that could have happened to me. It got me off my ass to start writing this book and the two blogs I have created. That made me feel good about myself for the first time in years.

In Buddhism, the first *Paramita* (perfection) that one should cultivate is that of *Dana.* Dana, or generosity, is encouraged as an essential attitude. This is the best way of offsetting the human tendency of individual self-centeredness and attachment.

But Suzuki, in *Zen Mind, Beginner's Mind* goes much further than that. Dana paramita is more than simple generosity. It comes from the realization that everything in the universe is one. As such, there is absolutely no reason to cling onto anything. You are the same as everything around you. As such, it is in your basic nature to be generous. Fear and ignorance confuse us into thinking it's preferable to place one's self first in the scheme of things.

It is this pointless "clinging" that Buddhism tells us is at the root of our suffering.

In chapter 13 of the *Tao Te Ching,* Lao Tzu puts it plainly:

> *What is meant by saying that the greatest*
> *trouble is the strong sense of individual*
> *self that people carry in all*
> *circumstances?*

People are beset with great trouble
because they define their lives so
narrowly.

If they forsake their narrow sense of self
and live wholly, then what can they call
trouble?

Therefore, only one who dedicates himself
to the wholeness of the world is fit to tend
the world.

Only one who relinquishes the self can be
entrusted with the responsibility for the
life of the world.

Dana paramita, according to Suzuki, is "tending to the world" in Lao Tzu's meaning. This means doing the best you can for all beings without exception. That includes you, but in no greater way than for everything else.

Suzuki says that each of us has two minds. The "big" mind and the "little" mind. The little mind is the mind that keeps us going as organisms. Without it, we wouldn't survive. The big mind is the unitary mind of the universe. It is this mind that Lao Tzu is speaking of in his final paragraph of the book.

One of whole virtue is not occupied with
amassing material goods.

Yet, the more he lives for others, the richer
his life becomes.

The more he gives, the more his life
abounds.

The subtle truth of the universe is
beneficial, not harmful.

The nature of an integral being is to
extend virtue to the world unconditionally,
and to contend with no one.

Suzuki goes on to explain that we all can tell when the big mind is working within us. That's where creativity in us comes from. Creativity is one of the great paradoxes in the Western "cause and effect" metaphysics. We are forced to invent "black box" concepts like emergence and complexity to explain it.

But black boxes don't really explain anything. They merely identify and give a word to a phenomenon which we are clueless about.

Buddhism has no such problem. Human creativity is seen as the same creativity behind the big bang and the emergence of stars, planets and galaxies out of the sea of undifferentiated plasma that first existed. Not a *resulting* creativity, the *same* creativity.

If you have any doubts about our having two minds, Suzuki poses a question to you. "Why is it that it feels so much better to give to someone than to get?" I had never thought of that, and though it's an unproven assumption, I've never met anyone who felt differently.

The reason it feels good is that it is the big mind that is doing it…

That truth can be extended to any act of altruism which we may do. It always "feels" *right*.

The latest attempt by Western science to explain altruism is that morality is somehow encoded in our genes. Maybe so. Maybe it's just the result of survival of the fittest *group*. But diehard Darwinists deny that that even exists. How can it? Individual survival is what is key to passing on genes, not group survival.

Buddhism has no such problems. Forgive me, but it simply makes more sense to me than the Western view. Buddhism doesn't answer all the mysteries, but it doesn't create any new ones either.

Well and good. What's this got to do with ayahuasca and Barack Obama?

The title of this book is "Placebo." My whole idea was to try to cure myself with the placebo effect by using psychedelics to temporarily delude myself into thinking I'd been cured. In order to accomplish this, I'd need to give up the next three months of my life concentrating on *myself*.

That always felt a bit selfish and wrong. I "rationalized" it by telling myself that if I was going to be any use to the world I'd have to cure myself first. But that simply isn't true.

Sixteen years ago, in what I refer to as my idealism's "last hurrah," I volunteered to work to elect Ross Perot for six months. (Never mind how it came out in the end.) My position was the head of the West coast's Jewish support.

I've been a supporter of Obama since before he even announced he was running. In a later chapter I'll go into more detail on this. But as a supporter, I sent the campaign a little money and nothing else.

I comforted myself by saying that my son Barak would carry the torch for me this time. The truth is I had lost all sense of confidence and self respect over the last decade. I just didn't believe I could do much to help, and was *way* too worried about my health to bother anyway.

What was it Bob said?

> *You are a rationalizer who makes*
> *elaborate excuses and tries to talk*
> *themselves and others into believing what*
> *you dearly wish was true.*

I dearly wished that I could cure this disease and used my cure as an excuse not to rejoin the living. Although he meant to accomplish something else with his email, Bob woke me up to the wrongheadedness of my approach.

There can be no "cure" for me without *dana paramita*. I know that now. I'm still an idealist, if a bit battered and bruised with time.

The greatest good to the greatest number of beings on the planet will result if Obama gets elected. As far as I'm concerned, he's the last chance we've got of holding the US together… At least over the short term.

So I choose to work full time towards accomplishing that goal. Big mind versus little mind. There's no contest for me.

In terms of the placebo effect, maybe instead of deluding myself with psychedelics into thinking I'm cured, I'll rely on the "big mind" to save me. If I contribute enough, I might even start believing that it's curing me and I'll enable the placebo effect just the same.

Last Saturday I spent Shabbat with our local *Chabad* rabbi who's a friend of mine. We had long discussions comparing Jewish mysticism with Buddhism. It was a wonderful time for me. He's a great guy to talk with.

In any event, at one point he pointedly asked me, "What is it that you want?!"

A difficult question to answer…

After thinking it over for a while, when I thought of the answer I *knew* it was right.

"I want to have a clear conscience…"

Part Two

LDN – Miracle Cure Found!

22. Miracle Cure?

It's hard for me to believe it myself. For the last month or so I have been *symptom free!*

1. No urinary urgency...
2. No balance problems...
3. No memory problems...
4. No ADD problems...

Huh?!!!!!

If I had confidence that it would continue, it would certainly qualify as the "miracle cure" I have been seeking.

What seems to have brought this state of affairs about (believe it or not) is my own research into medications, combined with my planning for the aborted ayahuasca treatment.

I had been waiting for two months for UCSF to get its act together regarding the Tysabri treatment. In the meantime I had started taking a treatment called LDN (Low dose Naltrexone).

When I went to ask for the Tysabri, I also asked my doctor if I could try the LDN. I had found out about it online when searching for the best MS specialist on the west coast who turned out to be Dr Goodin at

UCSF. At the UCSF website there was a little box saying they had completed a "patient funded" study of the effects of LDN on Multiple Sclerosis.

When I asked Dr. Goodin about the study he shrugged and said he hadn't expected any results from it, but in fact the limited eight week study had shown some results.

I asked him if I should try taking that too. He replied that it couldn't hurt and wrote me out a prescription for it. I asked him about potential conflicts with the Tysabri. He snorted and laughed, "It's 4.5 mg, about the size of a pin head. It won't conflict with anything."

Because of the nonchalant way that Dr. Goodin had spoken of it I had expected nothing from it. I started taking it the way one takes vitamins. A vague hope that maybe it might help in some indefinable way.

Naltrexone is a drug used to help recovering addicts. The only dosage manufactured is 50 mg, so I had to find a compounding pharmacy to make up the 4.5 mg dosage that the treatment called for.

Because of the long delay in getting the Tysabri, I decided to wait until after Peru before beginning it. It involves a massive infusion once a month in a hospital. The thinking was that it was best to avoid mixing other chemicals in my body during the ayahuasca sessions in order to avoid potential bad interactions.

Tysabri is considered a second line treatment for MS. Although it has by far the best track record of reducing relapses (67% reduction as opposed to 30% for the other approved treatments), one needs to get special dispensation in order to get it.

This is because Tysabri appears to interact with other immune-modulating drugs to cause progressive multifocal leukoencephalopathy (PML), an often-fatal opportunistic viral infection.

I had been willing to take the risk, though. I couldn't continue down the path I was on.

The other research I did was looking for a replacement for the Provogil. Although it made me feel more awake, it did nothing for my ADD symptoms. Additionally, I needed 400 mg a day of the stuff and I was concerned about potential interactions with the ayahuasca.

I began searching for a drug that would give me the most "bang for the buck" in terms of effectiveness for the dose. That was when I discovered Desoxyn.

This was the line in Wikipedia that convinced me to try and get it.

> *Further, because the secondary effects of dextromethamphetamine hydrochloride (Desoxyn) are least among the amphetamine-class stimulants or methylphenidate but the highest degree of primary effectiveness (i.e., most effective at enhancing concentration and decreasing distractibility, with the least occurrence of side effects), Desoxyn can be useful for patients who find other medications ineffective or for whom the side effects of such other medications are too severe.*

Apparently, one needed to take three times the amount of Dexedrine to get the same effect as that provided by Dysoxyn.

My doctor did not feel qualified to prescribe it so I went to a psychiatrist who treats people with ADD. He had never even *heard* of the drug, but after reading up on it, agreed to give me a two weeks supply as a trial.

The bottom line? As a result of preparing for the ayahuasca cure, I ended up on LDN and Desoxyn and *nothing else.* I've now been on LDN for about 4 months and Desoxyn for about a month and a half.

I never expected the LDN to affect my ongoing symptoms. I was taking it on the off chance that it could help reduce my chances of a relapse. But one day I noticed I needed to pee and when I went to the bathroom I was amazed… It kept coming and coming!

Thinking it over, I realized that I hadn't had to pull over to the side of the road to relieve myself for a long time. How long had it been? Two weeks... A month... WOW!!!

I couldn't believe my luck! It was the last thing I had anticipated. Thinking it over, I realized that I hadn't had any real balance problems lately either. Was it possible the LDN had taken care of both symptoms? I could think of nothing else that could have helped.

If LDN is that effective at such tiny doses with *zero* side effects, why isn't it the FIRST drug that is prescribed for MS? Clearly I was not the first person it had helped, but it wasn't even recognized by the FDA as being a legitimate treatment for MS.

My God... There could only be one answer that made any sense. The pharmaceutical industry!

Here's what Wikipedia says:

> *Low dose naltrexone (LDN), where the drug is used in doses approximately one-tenth those used for drug/alcohol rehabilitation purposes, is being used by some as an "off-label" experimental treatment for certain immunologically-related disorders, including HIV/AIDS, multiple sclerosis* [6] *Parkinson's, cancer, autoimmune diseases such as rheumatoid arthritis or ankylosing spondylitis, and central nervous system disorders.*

What they fail to mention is that naltrexone has been out of patent for 20 years or so. It's available as a generic and even with the special compounding required, a four month supply cost me $25 copay.

The Copaxone injections, that I had been using when first diagnosed, cost $1,500 for a month's supply. I had to stop the Copaxone after two months because each daily injection would leave behind a painful cyst that remained for three weeks. It was simply intolerable.

The Tysabri would have cost around $3,000 a month. I would have needed to keep taking either of those drugs for the rest of my life.

Ask yourself, if you were a drug company which would you rather sell? LDN at $10 a month or Tysabri at $3,000 a month?

Before the internet, there would have been no way at all for me to even find out about the existence of LDN. As it is, it is never even mentioned on most of the MS sites. It is never mentioned as a treatment on a par with the standard ones.

The Copaxone I had tried to use was one of the standard treatments for MS. The other main drug used for MS is Interferon. I had chosen Copaxone over Interferon because the main side effect of the Interferon is flu-like symptoms. Who the hell wants that?

As I mentioned earlier, the Tysabri has been linked to fatalities from PML. Wikipedia lists its common side effects as fatigue and allergic reactions with a low risk of anaphylaxis (severe life threatening allergic reaction) headache, nausea, and colds.

Given that it works without any side effects, why isn't LDN the obvious *FIRST CHOICE* for treatment of MS?

The excuse given is that the evidence supporting LDN is merely "anecdotal," never having been properly tested. Anybody want to guess as to why no tests have been done on it?

All of us have read about how the pharmaceutical industry is interested in making money rather than actually helping patients. Now I was experiencing it firsthand!

As big as a surprise as the LDN was for me, the Desoxyn was and equal shock.

Within a few days of substituting 10 mg of it for the 400 mg of Provogil I had been using, I was back to a *fully functioning* brain. After two weeks and raising the dose to 25 mg a day I can honestly say that I haven't felt or functioned better for as long as I can remember. At least ten, maybe fifteen years.

1. No more getting lost in town...
2. No more forgetting everything...
3. No more daily exhaustion at 5 PM...
4. No more technophobia...

It seemed like every symptom not handled by the LDN was *knocked out of the ballpark* by the Desoxyn.

Originally I had asked for the Provogil because I wanted to avoid amphetamine based drugs. All of us have heard about the problems caused by "speed." Its illicit use has been labeled an "epidemic" in the US by the press.

We're all are so scared of methamphetamine that when I asked on the Patients Like Me forum whether anyone had tried using it to treat MS related ADD symptoms, I was almost banned from the site. All sorts of ignorant, hysterical attacks on me. And this was just for *asking* about it...

The reason I had asked was that no one there knew anything about Desoxyn.

I don't want to be addicted to anything. I don't want to be turned into a toothless, manic scarecrow. I don't want to have to use more and more of a drug to have it be effective.

All of the above are what we have been taught to expect from amphetamines. Undoubtedly it happens to some people who get hooked on the stuff. What I didn't know was that when used by people who actually need it, it has no such side effects. Wikipedia again:

> *As with other amphetamines, the majority of these side-effects are uncommon in therapeutic use, with the exception of growth retardation in children. Desoxyn also has a higher benefit relative to the*

incidence of side-effects than other amphetamines.

So the bottom line with Desoxyn is that no one uses it because of false fears generated as a side effect of the government's war on *some* drugs.

This is really OUTRAGEOUS if you think about it. All my symptoms from MS were made to vanish by two readily available drugs. Few MS sufferers know anything about either of them. They go on spending thousands of dollars a month on drugs with severe side effects that don't work as well.

I have got to get this information out to everyone... Talk about *dana paramita*!

Just in time too... I had been planning on volunteering full time for Barak Obama, but after his betrayal on FIMA I've been unable to work up any real enthusiasm for it.

A chance to *really* help a lot of people out there has just been handed to me on a silver platter.

It also has handed me a real reason to finish and promote this book. After deciding not to do the ayahuasca cure, I thought that the book was probably going to die on the vine. The main interest of my target audience would have been in the psychedelic/spiritual aspect of my "miracle cure."

Now, though the "cure" I accidentally discovered may be prosaic, it is available easily and for much less money than what MS sufferers are currently paying for drugs that have needless, awful side effects.

That is potentially *much* more helpful than anything I could have discovered with the ayahuasca.

So as a result of Bob's blowing me off, instead of losing my chance for a miracle cure, I discovered a cure that was right there all along. There's the twofold bonus of having a new raison d'être for this book as well as a raison d'être for me.

Lao Tzu summed up my circumstances in chapter 58 of the Tao Te Ching:

> *Disaster is what blessing perches on.*
> *Blessing is where disaster abides.*
> *Who can say what the ultimate end of all*
> *possibilities will be?*
> *Appropriate means soon become unfitting.*
> *Good means soon turn to evil.*

23. How did this happen?

The first serendipitous event that led to my discovery that LDN could stop Progressive Relapsing Multiple sclerosis stands out from the rest. This was about a month after my watch was "on too tight."

I was sitting out on the rattan swing outside my office. It was my favorite place to listen to lecture series on my Ipod. Where we live, Bonny Doon outside of Santa Cruz is a mountainous area covered with Redwood trees.

I would stretch out for hours at a time, the swing barely moving. While listening, I got to soak in maybe 200 varieties of lush plants that cover every available centimeter of ground. I was right next to our sloping driveway and my favorite thing was to chuck my still smoldering cigarette butts onto it without having to bother to stub them out first.

I guess it was my way of feeling "wicked" at the time, which shows you just how thin my life had become at that point. Naturally, I would sweep them all up later, but it gave me a real sense of freedom to be able to flick my buts away without a care.

The cordless phone next to me in the swing rang. I fumbled to pause the Ipod and answered.

I couldn't believe the sound that came out. "Joe?"

I instantly recognized the voice, "Oh my god, Dianne?"

Diane Fenner had been my girlfriend for about four years in college and law school. We had almost, but not quite, gotten married. I had not heard her voice in over 20 years, but there are some sounds one never forgets.

"It's been... How long, more than 20 years for sure? Why are you calling me now?"

"I don't know... I just felt like it."

She wanted to catch up on what had happened in my life. I took a deep breath.

"I'm sorry Diane, I've had the luckiest life one could ask for; it's just that I've recently been diagnosed with Relapsing Remitting MS."

I went on to explain that it wasn't the MS that was worrying me at the moment but the operation I had scheduled in 10 days to replace part of my neck with a titanium frame and some dead guy's bone material.

Because my afflicted left arm has no reflexes rather than the hyper reflexes associated with MS, my neurologist believed it was being caused by the spinal compression that showed up in the MRI, rather than the MS which had shown up as lesions on both my brain and spinal cord.

"I don't do well in operations, Diane. The last one I had almost killed me."

I was referring to the abdominal surgery I had had in Los Angeles to sever "adhesions" left from an unnecessary appendectomy I had had at Hadassah hospital in Jerusalem at the age of 17.

My problems with the medical profession go way back...

She sounded a bit crestfallen by the news. I tried to cheer her up by describing all the wonderful things about my life in Bonny Doon. How incredibly peaceful it was... How we didn't even have a key to lock the house... How my kids didn't even know what danger was... etc.

"I don't get it. But what have you been *doing*?" She wanted to know.

The truth of the matter was that I hadn't really *done* anything in the 7 years since 9/11 when I got hit with the depression. The depression had been augmented by a long bout with panic attacks that had rendered me effectively useless.

At the time, after I figured out what was happening to me, I had assumed it was just a reaction to the natural fear prompted by the attacks. I had left Israel 5 years earlier to get as far away from Islamic insanity as I could. The anthrax business had hit me the hardest.

There I was, in the safest, most remote place imaginable and I was scared to death to get my mail out of the mail box. I used surgical gloves handling it and would stand by the outside garbage to slice out only the necessary interiors of the mail I *knew* I needed. The junk mail and the envelopes went straight into the can.

After months of this, and months of talk-talk therapy, my therapist gave up and told me to go to an MD to get chemical aid. I was given Prozac and Xanax and managed to finally get the symptoms down to a tolerable level. But a deeper damage had remained.

Since that time, I was unable to function properly. I spent all my time studying philosophy and science. My wife was making us money on the internet. I was content to retreat to my world of abstract thinking and avoid *anything* real. The first half of this book demonstrates precisely the kind of things I absorbed myself in.

I had become your classic *luftmenchin,* (Yiddish – lit. "flying man").

Diane couldn't make any sense out of what I told her. She remembered me most as epitomizing the Billy Joel song "Angry Young Man." For good reason. Chairman of SDS at Columbia College. Joining the Israeli Navy after finishing Columbia Law School. The list goes on and on.

Diane knew me as an idealistic man of action. The bemused, gentle scholar she was speaking to now just didn't fit. I defended myself. I thought I had grown past that stage in my life. Age and wisdom had taught me the essential pointlessness of my old patterns and I was much happier this way, I explained.

She didn't buy it, but all of a sudden she grew quiet.

"Wait a minute… I don't BELIEVE this!" She almost shouted.

"What are you talking about?"

"I just remembered…" Her voice grew serious and hurried. "The very first case I won after finishing law school concerned a woman who had your exact same diagnoses."

Diane had been studying for her PHD in psychology when we had broken up. She had gotten the degree, but after a short time working in the field had decided that it was a dead end. She then went to law school, got her JD and had since become a very successful lawyer who specialized in lawsuits against drug companies.

The case she was remembering concerned a woman who had been diagnosed with the identical spinal condition that my MRI showed. It had some 14 syllable, unpronounceable name which she pronounced with ease. It had resulted in the exact same "dead arm" symptom that I was suffering from.

The woman was told she needed the same operation that I was scheduled for (another unpronounceable string of syllables). After the operation, they realized that in fact she had MS. The stress to her body from the operation caused her to have a major relapse. She had walked into the hospital, and had come out in a wheelchair.

"Joe, they didn't even go to deposition. They just caved and paid. It was that open and shut."

Not that different from my case, I thought, though I had already been diagnosed as having both conditions. But this news reminded me of a great truth that in my fear and suffering I had forgotten…

Doctors are HUMAN. They make MISTAKES. What if they were wrong and my dead arm was being caused not by the spinal compression but by the MS? I could end up like that first client. Or maybe worse…?

"Damn…. I better think about this." I had been looking for an excuse to avoid the operation, and this was my chance. "Maybe I should see an MS specialist. I'll try and find the number one authority on the west coast. If *he* tells me my condition can't be caused by MS, I'll go ahead with the operation."

Diane was enthusiastic about this idea. So was I. The operation loomed over me as a possible death sentence. This gave me hope for a commutation.

So I followed up on this conversation that fell on me out of the blue after more than 20 years. I began researching to find this mythical "number one specialist" on the west coast. It didn't take me that long to find him.

Here's the listing for him at UCSF:

Douglas Goodin, M.D.
Medical director, Multiple Sclerosis Center

Dr. Douglas Goodin, director of the Multiple Sclerosis Center at UCSF Medical Center, is a neurologist and an internationally renowned expert in the treatment and research of multiple sclerosis.. He earned a bachelor of sciences degree in genetics and biochemistry at the University of Washington in Seattle; a master of sciences degree in molecular biology at Purdue University in Indiana; and a medical degree from the University of California, Irvine. He completed a residency in neurology at UCSF where he joined the medical center staff in 1982. In addition to multiple sclerosis, Goodin's

research interests include various forms of
dementia. Goodin also is a professor of
neurology at UCSF.

I noticed in a little side box a mention that a "patient funded study" had
been done on the effects of LDN on multiple sclerosis. In the box, it
said that the study had been completed, but it had no mention of the
results. I had never heard of a "patient funded study" before, and I made
a mental note to ask Goodin what the results had been, and thought no
more about it.

When I got in to see Goodin, a few days before the scheduled operation,
I asked him, "If you tell me my dead arm couldn't be caused by the MS
I'll have the operation."

"I can't tell you that," he replied, "In fact I think it *is* being caused by
the MS?"

"What about it having *no* reflexes instead of hyper reflexes?"

He answered that though hyper reflexes are usually the case, MS can
sometimes cause no reflexes as well.

Utterly relieved, I canceled the operation. I also noted to myself what
makes an expert.

Experts know all the *exceptions* to the rule as well as the rule.

I forgot to ask about the LDN box on the website as it was decided that I
should begin on the copaxone.

In April, a little more than two months later, I began to panic after the
major cognitive problems began to emerge. I also decided I had to give
up the copaxone because of the horrible reactions I was having at every
injection site.

I went back to Dr. Goodin and had the exchange described in the
previous chapter.

The almost "afterthought" way in which he treated the LDN made me think that there was nothing much to expect from it. I'd take it because there was nothing to lose, even though there wasn't much to expect, either.

A month later, the cognitive problems continued to worsen. I began to do research on line in earnest. The kinds of problems I was having should not be caused by the small number of lesions that had shown up on my MRI.

I came across three abstracts that described the characteristics of people with the rare form of MS, progressive relapsing. These included being male, being older, and having "spinal atrophy." Most MS patients are female and are diagnosed before turning 40.

I didn't know what "spinal atrophy" meant, but when I returned to UCSF to present them with this possible diagnosis I found out it was just a fancy word for the spinal compression that had almost gotten me another unnecessary operation.

After the usual resistance to listening to anything a patient might contribute to his own diagnoses, the doctor there sadly agreed that PRMS was probably the best diagnosis. Unfortunately, since there was nothing that could be done for the progressive part of the MS, it was decided I should go ahead with the Tysabri to at least try to prevent relapses.

It was now June, and I was going to be off to Peru in another month. I finally get word that UCSF was ready to give me the Tysabri. I met with Grace, my GP, together with Bob and we decided it would be best to delay the Tysabri treatment until my return.

The concern was that no shaman could possibly know about the Tysabri and whether there might be conflicts with the ayahuasca.

Soon after that, Bob dumped me for having begun smoking again. I was forced to choose what I wanted to do and I chose the Buddhist *dana paramita* rather than the shaman approach. I would volunteer full time for Barack Obama.

When Obama failed to lead on the FISA issue, and instead caved in to the Republican talking points, I felt as if the rug had been pulled out from under my feet. I had already made contacts within the campaign and was preparing to spend my time up until the election convincing Jews in Florida to vote for Obama rather than McCain.

I talked it over with my son Barak. He said that though he felt Obama had made a serious mistake, there was still every reason to work for him. "Abba, this election is probably the most important election…" He paused and thought for a while before finishing, "Maybe *ever.*"

I knew he was right. The US was going into a major nose dive because of the catastrophic policies of the Bush administration. We were headed for some unavoidable *very* bad times no matter what. The only question was whether it could be turned around before it would destroy the foundation of the world as we knew it. Maybe Obama could do that much.

My problem was that I knew I simply couldn't get up in front of an audience and urge them to vote for a candidate for whom I felt less than total enthusiasm.

A few days later all my symptoms disappeared.

So here's what's needed to have happened for me to have found out what I found out about LDN.

1. Diane needed to call after 20 years to stop the operation.
2. UCSF needed to have done the LDN study for me to have heard of it.
3. Goodin needed to be flip about LDN or I might have researched it and had high hopes. That could have raised the issue of the placebo effect in my cure.
4. I needed to have had horrible cognitive problems to figure out I had PRMS.
5. UCSF had to have bureaucratic problems to allow for the Tysabri delay.
6. I needed to be planning to do the ayahuasca, or I would have begun the Tysabri.
7. Bob had to blow me off for smoking.

8. I needed an Obama-like focus to decide to try *dana paramita* rather than the ayahuasca.
9. The symptoms had to disappear when they did or I would have credited the Tysabri rather than the LDN.

On July 16, I realized that the greatest chance at *dana paramita* has just been handed to me on a silver platter.

> On my blog I receive the following comment:
>
> Dear Joe,
>
> As editor/owner of http://www.ldninfo.org I was delighted to see your fervent message. Someone who has not only experienced LDN but also is a gifted writer is a real find! We're counting on you to tell the world.
>
> As a retired internist, my personal hope is that once we can point to a few convincing medical journal articles (at least two more are due this year), we should be able to jump all over the health-related committees of Congress to force them to modify the current damaging system of approvals run by Big Pharma and take advantage of LDN's enormous possibilities for the public's health.
>
> Regards,
>
> David Gluck, MD

Unbelievable… The "miracle cure" that I was going to try to find in Peru was available at the corner drug store for about a dollar a day.

It is a cliché and a truism, I know. But I have just experienced the fact that the greatest "miracles" of life often manifest as mundane routine.

It feels as though because I was searching for something to do for the world as a way to find my cure, my cure was handed to me as a way to help the world.

I'll never stop being a rationalist, but there are some weird things that happen in life that we can't or maybe shouldn't ignore. I feel like I *owe*.

This book is no longer a journal of a desperate man. It has become a call to arms to spread the word of how LDN can help not only MS sufferers like me, but also all people suffering from any immune system disorder.

That's an awful lot of people. I hope I'm up to the task. It's so big, with such enormous consequences that it makes me wonder again about my sanity. Grandiose ideas rarely lead to anything other than disappointment.

My first attempts to get the word out on my MS support forums have met with mixed success. The pharmaceutical companies have clearly loaded the forums with reps to push their expensive and ineffective treatments. I have been repeatedly and viciously attacked for trying to get the info out.

Not all the responses have been like that, for sure, but enough have been that way to make me understand that it is not going to be easy for me to spread this truth that was dropped on me from I know not where.

There are literally billions of dollars at stake here that are not going to be surrendered without a fight.

But at least I'm not alone. Another book, *The Promise of Low Dose Naltrexone: Potential Benefits for Cancer, Autoimmune, Neurological and Infectious Disorders,* by health writer Elaine A. Moore and LDN Advocate SammyJo Wilkinson, was published in December, 2008. It's a book intended for physicians with all the scientific evidence to back up trying LDN.

I intend to try to get this book out for Christmas. With two books being promoted and the new studies getting published, it's at least possible Dr. Gluck's plan to pressure Congress will come to something.

I haven't been involved in a "fight" for a long, long time. The last big one was volunteering to return to Israel from LA to fight with my old Navy unit in the first Gulf War.

This time it will be somewhat different. I will try to use what I have learned during my illness to help me make the "fight" not a fight at all.

During the times to come I will try to use as my guide Lao Tzu's *Tao Te Ching.*:

> *The sage does not distinguish between*
> *himself and the world;*
> *The needs of other people are as his own.*
>
> *He is good to those who are good;*
> *He is also good to those who are not good,*
> *Thereby he is good.*
> *He trusts those who are trustworthy;*
> *He also trusts those who are not*
> *trustworthy,*
> *Thereby he is trustworthy.*
>
> *The sage lives in harmony with the world,*
> *And his mind is the world's mind.*
> *So he nurtures the worlds of others*
> *As a mother does her children.*

24. Snake Oil or Penicillin for the Immune System?

The main Yahoo support group for LDN users is called lowdosenaltrexone, It has over five thousand members and receives over a thousand posts a month. It is managed by the same people who run the biggest LDN website, www.lowdosenaltrexone.org.

On the main page of the group is the following description:

> About LDN: FDA-approved naltrexone, in a low dose, can boost the immune system — helping those with HIV/AIDS, cancer, autoimmune diseases, and central nervous system disorders.

> In May 2006, clinical trial researchers at Pennsylvania State University College of Medicine reported: "LDN therapy offers an alternative safe, effective, and economic means of treating subjects with active Crohn's disease."

> Other physicians and researchers have described beneficial effects of LDN on a variety of diseases, including Multiple Sclerosis (MS), Pancreatic Cancer, HIV/AIDS, ALS (Lou Gehrig's Disease), Autism Spectrum Disorders, Behcet's Disease, Irritable Bowel Syndrome (IBS), Parkinson's Disease, Psoriasis, Rheumatoid Arthritis, Systemic Lupus (SLE), and Wegener's Granulomatosis.

When I first saw this, my heart sank. What had I hitched my horse to? Another "new age cure-all" cure nothing fad? How could any drug be effective in helping so many different diseases that seemed, on the face of it, to have nothing to do with one another?

Mind you, I *knew* it had relieved me of all my MS symptoms… But autism and psoriasis? Give me a break! These had to be wild unsubstantiated ravings of wishful thinkers. No drug can do so much good for so many illnesses. It had to be bull…

I began searching my memory for any other drug in medical history that had ever done that much good for so many diseases. After a while I came up with only one other such example… *penicillin*

> *The discovery of penicillin marked a turning point in history and dramatically changed the impact of medicine. It is hard to comprehend now the fear that arose from even a minor infection, as treatment often required the lancing of swollen glands and sometimes amputation, in an attempt to save the patient's life. Death from even minor infections was common. The advent of penicillin changed not only the course of medicine, but of society as well, as it permitted physicians to prescribe a medication that could save lives within a few days of its administration.*

> http://www.encyclopedia.com/doc/1G1-143440246.html

What made penicillin so different from all previous drugs was that it seemed to work on just about *every* kind of infection that routinely sickened and killed millions of people a year.

What was it about penicillin that made it so remarkably effective?

> Penicillin is an antibiotic that destroys Bacteria by destroying the cell wall of the microorganism. It does this by inactivating an enzyme necessary for the cross linking of bacterial cell walls. The enzyme is known as transpeptidase. It accepts the penicillin as a substrate, it then alkanolates nucleophilic oxygen of the enzyme, rendering it inactive. Cell wall construction stops and the bacteria soon die. The antibiotic nature of the penicillin is due to the strained b-lactam ring, on opening the ring strain is relieved this makes penicillin more reactive than ordinary amides.

http://wiki.answers.com/Q/How_does_penicillin_work_in_the
_human_body

The operant phrase here is *"destroys Bacteria."* Not one particular disease's bacteria, but *bacteria* period. That's what made it effective against so many catastrophic illnesses that harmed and killed so many people a year.

It's now known that evolutionary processes have produced bacteria that are resistant to penicillin, but for many years the drug was a guaranteed cure-all for any and all infectious diseases.

In order to begin to believe the incredible claims being made by the proponents of LDN, it is necessary to understand the way the drug actually produces the effects it is claimed to produce.

Why LDN is Effective in MS and Other Autoimmune Disorders

low dose haltrexone works to modulate the immune system and help the body heal itself. By increasing the production of endorphins, which act as neurotransmitters, modulating immune function, low dose naltrexone helps the body return to a state of homeostasis and heal itself.

Rather than being overactive, the immune system cells in autoimmune disease are weak and ineffective. Once the immune system has been strengthened, courtesy of LDN use, the normalized immune system stops its "illegal" attack on the body's own cells, thus halting any further progression of the autoimmune disorder.

In fact, administration of LDN *triples* the body's production of endorphins. You could run for 24 hours a day and not get that kind of endorphin boost. Only recently has the effect of endorphins on the immune system been recognized. But recognized it has been. A Google search for "endorphins immune system" produced **414,000** results.

The bottom line is that the reason LDN is so effective against so many diseases is that our immune systems are effective against so many diseases. We have millions of years of evolutionary selection behind us to protect us against most diseases, but especially diseases that are caused by our own body malfunctioning. All LDN does is strengthen our bodies' protections against these illnesses. It doesn't affect the illness itself.

So how is this like penicillin? On one level it's not like it at all. Penicillin directly attacks the bacteria which cause the illness. On another level it's quite similar in that it affects *all* diseases related to a weakened or malfunctioning immune system, the way penicillin affects *all* diseases caused by bacteria.

It's this level of similarity that gives LDN the "snake oil effect." It works on so many diseases that it's hard to believe it's for real.

Pretty much every person I have tried to tell about the effects of LDN has had the same reaction I did at first. When told of the number of diseases it can help, most of them diseases known to have no real cure available, I get the skeptical "You gotta be kidding me..." response.

Doctors are no exception to this rule. They have to put up with umpteen numbers of new age "snake oil" cures that their patients eagerly try to convince them to adopt. The doctors have developed their own kind of "immune system" against such fraudulent cure-alls. It's hard to blame them from reacting to LDN the same way.

Except for the fact that there is now so much evidence out there that LDN works as its proponents claim, that one has to purposely turn a blind eye to the evidence available to anyone who bothers to search the internet.

Why would doctors, even good doctors, do such a thing?

First of all, the specialists who see these sorts of patients have had many years of medical training from which they become absolutely committed to accepting only the scientific evidence as presented in their favorite peer-reviewed medical journals.

Because LDN is out of patent, no one has invested the millions of dollars necessary to perform the sorts of trials that generally get published in these journals.

My own belief is that the main culprit preventing doctors from even considering LDN is the runaway malpractice epidemic that has swept the US over the last few decades. Ask your doctor, ask *any* doctor what his biggest expense is in running his practice and he will tell you it's malpractice insurance.

Naltrexone is an FDA approved drug for the treatment of recovering addicts. Using it for any other purpose, while legal, is considered "off label use." While there's nothing wrong with that per se, doctors have reason to fear that if something were to go wrong they could be easily sued. FDA approval for the treatment provided gives them a pretty rock solid defense. Off label use is something they would have to actually *prove* was the right thing to do.

So just as in government bureaucracies and in corporate hierarchies, *"ass covering"* is the name of the game. Of course this violates their Hippocratic Oath to the core. I believe that's one of the reasons it's so difficult to get a doctor to even *research* whether LDN would be the right treatment.

Like the statue we've all seen of the three monkeys: *See no evil, Hear no evil, Speak no evil.*

The evil for the doctors is malpractice suits.

Unfortunately for the patients, the evil they suffer is no relief for their horrendous affliction.

25. Google LDN!

Let's check on Google to see what the chances are of finding out about LDN's effects on the various diseases it is known to have a positive effect on. We'll begin with my own disease, Multiple Sclerosis.

The first listing Google returns is for the National Multiple Sclerosis Society at: *www.nmss.org/.* If one goes there to the "newly diagnosed" section and then clicks on "Understanding treatment options" one is presented with a box listing the "FDA Approved Treatments" which include: Avonex (interferon beta-1a),Betaseron (interferon beta-1b),Copaxone (glatiramer acetate),Novantrone (mitoxantrone),Rebif (interferon beta-1a),Tysabri (natalizumab).

All of these drugs have harsh or even fatal side effects and are not particularly good at stopping relapses and have absolutely no effect whatsoever on progressive MS.

At the bottom of the page, the last entry under "Treatment Updates" reads as follows:

Low Dose Naltrexone Update

Jun 02, 2008

We have received a number of inquiries about the use of low dose naltrexone (LDN) as a treatment for multiple sclerosis. There are currently no published data from controlled clinical trials to support the use of naltrexone

in MS. Further study is needed to determine if this is a
safe and effective treatment for people with MS.

Of course this is completely out of date as will be seen later on, and it
reflects the fact that this organization is utterly uninterested in LDN and
only posted what it posted because of the "number of inquiries" it
received.

Under the National Multiple Sclerosis Society entry, Google offers us a
chance to "Refine results for multiple sclerosis:" If one chooses
"Treatment," the first mention of LDN is at position 30. The problem is
that it is a link to the same page at the National Multiple Sclerosis
Society, mentioned above. The next time LDN shows up is at position
153 at:
  www.lowdosenaltrexone.org /ldn_and_ms.htm.

That means for most people who surf with Google's default of 10
returns per page they would have to go for 15 pages to get there.
Knowing my own habits, I rarely search further than 5 pages, figuring
anything important would be covered in that many returns.

In the Google listing itself for MS, LDN shows up as the 128th position
and it is the same good listing that showed up in the 153rd position under
"Treatment." This is actually a big improvement. A month ago the first
mention of LDN was at the 201st position. However, it still means that
one would have to go 12 pages deep in the search in order to find it.

LDN is the only drug known that stops Primary Progressive MS.
Remember, I was told at the best MS center on the west coast at UCSF
that there was *no* treatment available for it. So let's search for "primary
progressive multiple sclerosis PPMS."

Something actually showed up at the 29th position! But wait, that's new.
Published on September 18, 2008 at suite101.com the article focuses on
a recent test done in Italy that showed that LDN halted progression in
PPMS patients. (See appendix) In a little box at the top of the page
reads the following:

> Low dose naltrexone has been used in the
> treatment of multiple sclerosis for over 20

years, but only now was the first official study
published.

That actually isn't true. There have been plenty of studies done in the
past, just not many that were published in medical journals. The title of
the article is: *Low Dose Naltrexone: Hope for PPMS - New Trial of LDN
in Primary Progressive Multiple Sclerosis.*

The article reports on the successes of the trial but includes the
following statement:

Study Results

> LDN markedly reduced spasticity, while
> pain, fatigue and depression did not
> improve (or improvement didn't reach
> statistical significance). The study did not
> evaluate urinary frequency, a common
> symptom of MS and often reportedly
> helped by LDN. It should be noted that
> LDN is not intended for symptom
> improvement, but to slow down illness
> progression, though some patients do
> experience symptom relief.

Where they came up with that last sentence from, I have no idea.
Symptom relief is the thing LDN is *most* noted for in MS. In my case it
relieved *all* of them. That it stops or slows the illness progression is
what makes it so *critical* in this version of MS. But it stops relapses in
people with Remitting Relapsing MS and relieves symptoms there too.

Alright, so let's check for the next hit on LDN under PPMS. It's at
position 237 and is from the largest LDN site on the web,
lowdosenaltrexone.org. This is also a significant improvement from a month
ago when it showed up at the 301st position.

That means that until about a month ago the *only drug known to help this
condition* could only be found if one surfed 30 pages deep into Google on the
subject.

Checking into my own special weird version of MS, "Progressive Relapsing MS, PRMS" there is a hit at position 58 from the site *www.ldners.org* , another of the largest LDN sites. It reports on a survey done among MS sufferers using LDN and their reports of its effectiveness. A month ago it was at position 83. This is the first and only time I'm aware of that LDN shows up in the first five pages of a Google search.

One of the other relatively common diseases that LDN has been shown to be most effective at helping is Crohn's Disease. Let's see how Google does on that. Wow! Google only would give me "1000 of about 2,740,000 for Crohn's disease" and LDN doesn't show up at all!

Searching for Crohn's disease and LDN produced 4,800 results. But none of them make into the top 1000 for Crohn's disease, which is all Google will return. That means it's literally *impossible* to find out about LDN for Crohn's unless one already knows about it.

If one refines one's search with Google for "treatment," LDN shows up at the 122nd position. But it's only an entry on a forum at technocrat.com and it forwards the reader to a dead link. No other mention of LDN shows up in the entire search.

Let's try HIV AIDS, the disease that was first discovered to be helped by LDN. Same result as with Crohn's. It doesn't appear in the first thousand entries. It also is completely absent from the results if one refines one's search under Google for "treatment."

AIDS was the first disease discovered to be helped by LDN back in the '80s by Dr. Bihari. It was only later discovered to be helpful in any immune system related disorder.

A search for "HIV AIDS ldn" produced *79,000* hits!

How is it possible with that many hits that not even *one* of them shows up in the first 1000 Google hits, or anywhere at all under "treatment"?

Once again, if you don't know the acronym "LDN" you'll never find out from Google how it can help AIDS.

There's a definite pattern emerging here...

One that makes me wonder if someone isn't pulling strings somewhere to affect the search engine's results.

Let's end with a search for the most common of diseases that LDN is known to help, cancer.

There are so many sub variants of cancer that it's impossible to try to search them all out. I'll begin with cancer itself and then look into Multiple Myeloma, a disease that killed my friend 5 years ago.

A search for cancer on Google produces no hits on LDN in the first thousand sites which is all Google gives one access too. It also fails to show up anywhere under the "treatment" refined search.

This despite the fact that a search for "cancer ldn" produced **356,000** *hits.*

Same story for Multiple Myeloma. If you search for the disease by itself, you won't find any mention of LDN on Google. Searching for "Multiple Myeloma LDN" produced 3900 results.

Now you can understand why I decided to name this book, *"Google LDN !"* If you don't already know about it, there is virtually *no* chance of finding out about it using the most trusted and powerful search engine known.

That means you are stuck with what your doctor recommends, and as already discussed, it is highly unlikely that he or she will ever mention LDN.

How is this possible?

The facts about LDN's effect on immune system related diseases were discovered back in the 80s!

26. Reverse Search Engine Optimization (SEO)

Is it possible that the pharmaceutical industry with its nearly unlimited access to funds and a notorious history of business abuses could be behind LDN's no-show on Google?

Reverse SEO is the process of removing (technically pushing down) websites other than your own from the first pages of Google. There are two varieties of techniques referred to as "black hat" and "white hat."

If I were a pharmaceutical company seeking to preserve its billion dollar profits being made from drugs that compete with LDN, I would certainly consider using any and all of the following tactics.

Google Bowling is an example of a "black hat" technique used to lower another site's ranking.

Google Bowling - reverse SEO

Posted on Wednesday 4 July 2007

What is an SEO going to do when a certain competitor ranks better and it seems impossible to catch up with him? He'll either increase his regular SEO efforts even more, or think about using black hat SEO. Lately, a black hat SEO technique called "**Google Bowling**" has attracted the attention of the SEO community.

What is "Google Bowling" aka "reverse SEO"?

"**Google Bowling**," also called "**reverse SEO**" is a technique, based on the simple fact that there is a second way of getting on top of the Google search results:

- increasing your own rank
- **decreasing your competitor's rank**

Google Bowling is an SEO technique that is capable of **decreasing a competitor's rank in the Google Search Engine**

How does "Google Bowling" aka "reverse SEO" work?

Is it really possible to decrease a competitor's rank without touching his website? - Yes it is possible.

Google Bowling exploits the **ranking penalty algorithms** that Google applies to websites that are playing against the rules by **spamming other websites with inbound links**.

To bowl a website from the top of the Google results, an opponent needs to **spam** a huge amount of **other websites with links** to the target website in a short amount of time, to trigger Google's Anti-Spam algorithms. If the efforts are successful, Google will think that the target website is trying to illegitimately increase their rankings through spamming and apply a **ranking penalty** to that website, dropping it from the top search results or even making it completely disappear from the SERPS (Search Engine Result Pages).

Due to the huge amount of spam links needed for a **successful Google Bowl**, I believe that it is impossible to Google Bowl manually. From what I have heard, Google Bowling is mostly done with **automated website**

spamming software which targets forums or blogs with comment spam.

Is Google Bowling easy?

I haven't done Google Bowling myself and I am not planning to do it, but from what I have heard and from my knowledge about the Google Algorithms, it should not be an easy task due to the **huge amount of successful spam needed** within a short period of time.

Is Google Bowling legal? Should I try this?

No. **Do not try to Google bowl your competitors**. This is definitely an illegal activity and you might get sued for this. You have been warned…

http://optimized-promotion.com/seo/seo-classifications/black-hat-seo/google-bowling-reverse-seo.html

Here's another article describing "black hat" techniques for lowering your competitor's page ranking.

Reverse SEO: Kill The Competition And Fill The Void

Mon, 14 Apr 2008 09:57:37 by Joe Bursell

As competition in search continues to grow and grow, so to do the efforts of crooks and miscreants to hijack, damage or destroy the legitimately gained rankings of their competitors. We've seen many instances of malicious link insertion and now there are increasing examples of other attacks being used to tar the reputation of targeted websites.

If you can create a scenario in which your competitor's sites are seen by the search engines as hosting a bunch of spam/malicious links, your site can perform well in the void that is created. The techniques simply insert spam links into the target site. Once Google crawls that site and sees the spam it will see it is untrustworthy- once marked as spam the site may disappear altogether from the rankings.

This type of activity has been labeled "evil SEO," but that's way too simplistic a view. It is an attack, in the same way that defacement is an attack. What is interesting is that the value of search has reached such a peak that *any* method for gaining search visibility is worth a shot for some people.

So how would someone do this?..

...if a site allows the execution of mark-up or code inserted from a publicly accessible mechanism- such as through a browser- it is vulnerable. For example, if your site runs SQL it is possible that that someone can manipulate the site to insert content, in this case spammy links, or links to flagged malicious websites. This is most often achieved through the browser. If there is no filtering for certain characters, or if it allows the insertion of a string of characters where only numbers should go, then your site is vulnerable.

Similarly, with non-SQL web applications and sites it may be possible to insert mark-up or code into a form input field, or browser that will create on-page changes to a site- allowing it to be populated with spam links. This technique is often called XSS (cross-site scripting) by the SEO community, but it is more properly recognized as plain HTML Injection. For a basic discussion of XSS see the Wikipedia entry.

Increasingly, rivals are undermining each other's search engine optimization efforts and page rankings by

exploiting web application vulnerabilities to fool search engines into categorizing them as untrustworthy, or very low/zero authority. There is also plenty of evidence that social bookmarking sites are also used in attacks. One method is to spoof the IP of the target site (creating web traffic using their address, rather than your own).
Then bookmark a targeted page on their site using that spoofed IP. This can be done with multiple accounts, so it looks like the site is self-promoting on a grand scale. Once again trust, authority and rankings go out the window.

Of course security vulnerabilities are inevitable, but preventing many attacks can be achieved by building applications right, the first time round. Businesses need to know that the technologies they are using are not substantially flawed from the off, and suppliers and developers have a responsibility to implement secure code. This is cold comfort for those whose sites are vulnerable, and for who the costs of a code review or an application security test are out of reach- never mind any remediation work.

http://www.vertical-leap.co.uk/blog/Reverse-SEO-Kill-The-Competition-And-Fill-The-Void.asp

The following is from a web page promoting an SEO company. They pride themselves on using "white hat" as opposed to "black hat" methods of sabotaging a competitor. "Rip Off Reports" are just words used to describe the content that is being sought to be lowered in the search engine results.

Reverse SEO Strategy

As part of our SEO 2.0 process, our team of SEO specialists will focus on researching your website as well as the websites on the top five ranked pages on Google. We will target our SEO efforts to reducing the relevancy Google crawlers attribute to Rip Off Reports and other complaint forums. We will focus on optimizing these other websites organically by identifying keywords used to locate them to increase their ranking in Google, which will in turn push Rip Off Report ranking lower. We will also research keywords and apply inbound links to ensure that your site remains as the top listing in the Google.

Our SEO team also promises only to use the more ethical "whitehat" reverse SEO techniques; versus the less ethical "blackhat" techniques like building spammer sites and posting on Craigslist™, which may temporarily move a Rip Off Report down. Our Reverse SEO campaign uses the methods that Search Engine's look for and while blackhat techniques sometimes deliver temporary results, crawlers always recognize these tactics and penalize websites severely with much lower rankings for these practices.

The Following are our White-Hat tactics for Reverse SEO:

- Creating a Blog and Blogging about the keywords that appear in competitor's sites or Rip Off Reports.

  A blog will also create a platform to reference other sites and increase their ranking above Rip Off Report.

- Social Networking about your business

  We will make sure that your social networking campaign raises the ranking of the targeted sites while lowering the ranking of Rip Off Report. By identifying discussion forums, blogs, and bulletin boards for maximum effectiveness and relative to your industry we will post comments designed to cause Google's crawlers to return more favorable rankings to the targeted sites to degrade Rip Off Report's ranking.

- Press Releases including the keywords that appear in competitor's sites or Rip Off Reports.

  By distributing press releases to several internet press release and news sites that have been keyword optimized we will create additional pages to buffer between All your site and Rip Off Report. Good press releases can also lead to other media coverage which will lead to further sites about you appearing in the higher ranking pages of Google. Additionally, by optimizing your press release into the top ranking of Google and posting it to various other press release websites, we will provide another page that references your website to appear above Rip Off Report in the search engine results.

- Backlinks with Anchor Text with the keywords that appear in competitor's sites or Rip Off Reports.

  By backlinking relevant and high ranking sites we will cause Google's crawlers to assign a higher ranking to these targeted sites while reducing the relevancy to Rip Off Report and thus lower its ranking further.

  We will use these keywords as hyperlinks to various high relevancy websites, blogs, discussion boards and forums to improve their ranking and keep your ranking high and push Rip Off Report down in relevancy and ranking.

  http://www.searchenginepartner.com/First-page-placement/reverse-seo.html

The issue of reverse SEO is still out of the public's eye. People still trust the results they get from the search engines as reflecting the real ranking of the importance of the pages reported.

Clearly, nothing could be further from the truth!

An exasperated blogger summed up the situation as follows:

Let's face it; most of the large corporations are using very aggressive reverse SEO methods to bury the opinion of bloggers and others they fear. Why doesn't congress just let the corporations send squads of goons over to shut down any newspaper that dares to speak the truth? They are doing the same thing online right now, so why aren't they allowed to blockade the delivery gates at publishers and newspapers and be done with it??

http://blogs.computerworld.com/node/5770

27. What's to be done about all this?

LDN is caught up in a Catch 22 of sorts. The doctors won't prescribe it because there's no FDA approval. It can't get FDA approval because there's not enough money to be made from a generic drug to justify spending the millions of dollars necessary to get the FDA approval.

LDN is in the same virtual position as the "orphan drugs" that Congress passed special legislation in order to help.

From Wikipedia:

> In the U.S., an orphan drug is any drug developed under the Orphan Drug Act of January 1983 ("ODA"), a federal law concerning rare diseases ("orphan diseases"), defined as diseases affecting fewer than 200,000 people in the United States or low prevalence is taken as prevalence of less than 5 per 10,000 in the community.

> This has been adopted as a subclause of the Food and Drug Administration (FDA) regulations. The granting of orphan drug status is designed to encourage the development of drugs which are necessary but would be prohibitively expensive/unprofitable to develop under normal circumstances.

> Because medical research and development of drugs to treat such diseases is financially disadvantageous, companies that do so are rewarded with tax reductions and marketing exclusivity (a "monopoly")on that drug for an extended time (seven years post-approval).

If you enjoy irony, you'll *love* this.

LDN is exactly like an orphan drug in that it is prohibitively expensive to develop, i.e. pass FDA testing. The only reason it doesn't qualify as an "orphan drug" is that it concerns diseases that affect *millions* of people in the US.

So because it could help millions rather than thousands of Americans it doesn't qualify to get any help.

Huh?????????????

I know, it sounds completely absurd, but that's the way the law was written.

Nobody thought about a situation where a drug that has already gone generic would later be discovered to have *a much more important use than that for which it was originally developed.*

This country has stuck to its belief that the best way to develop new drugs and treatments is to leave it in the private sector and let the profit motive do its thing. In many ways, that has proven to be the right approach.

The US leads the world in new drug development.

Although the papers are filled with stories of rampant corrupt practices among the Big Pharma companies, there is little doubt that overall we are doing pretty well. Just considering how much life expectancy has increased in my lifetime is enough to convince me that we must be doing *something* right.

LDN represents a weird problem, but one that we can expect to occur more and more often as the number of drugs going generic increases and the continuing progress in using whatever is out there to help various medical conditions increases.

Remember aspirin? A generic headache reliever, it turned out to be one of the most effective ways of preventing heart attack and stroke.

From the American Heart Association:

> The American Heart Association recommends aspirin use for patients who've had a myocardial infarction (heart attack), unstable angina, ischemic stroke (caused by blood clot) or transient ischemic attacks (TIAs or "little strokes"), if not contraindicated. This recommendation is based on sound

evidence from clinical trials showing that aspirin helps prevent the recurrence of such events as heart attack, hospitalization for recurrent angina, second strokes, etc. (secondary prevention). Studies show aspirin also helps prevent these events from occurring in people at high risk (primary prevention).

Who could have anticipated this?

LDN is in the same position as aspirin was, except that it is not sold over the counter. As a result you need to convince a doctor to give you a prescription. A difficult task, as discussed earlier.

Clearly the government needs to tweak the system to deal with this problem that will only get worse with time.

Possible Solutions:

1. **Legislation extending the scope of the "Orphan Drug" law** to include those drugs out of patent for which new uses are discovered. This would reduce the requirements for approval and allow for government funding.

2. **An Institute of Medicine** [IOM] shall be empowered to become the health "czar," overseeing certain major decisions concerning all new medical treatments and devices. It may overrule the FDA when it deems necessary. The new IOM will be sufficiently funded and staffed to be able to arrange support for any and all necessary clinical trials it deems of value, and it shall choose those appropriate centers of excellence at which such studies shall be performed.

   (See appendix: *The US System to Develop Important Health Treatments at Low Cost is Being Hoodwinked*)

3. **Legislation to allow a substance to be "re-patented"** when a new use is discovered for it. Clearly, this would have to be limited to those substances which still required a prescription.

The advantage of this approach would be to bring the significant resources of the pharmaceutical industry to bear on new uses of old drugs as well as new drugs. It is also likely that the industry would actually support such a move rather than fight it, making its passage much more likely.

Among these three possible solutions, my favorite is the last. Like it or not, Big Pharma practically owns the congress. The chances of pushing through legislation that they oppose is unlikely if not impossible.

The other two solutions would be fought against tooth and nail by Big Pharma because they would both cause big dents in the potential profits that could be made.

I would much rather have big Pharma behind me than opposing me on the hill. My primary concern here is getting safe and effective drugs into the hands of people suffering, not who is making money out of the operation. Until the US joins the rest of the world in socializing its health care system, there really is no other choice.

Under the new system, LDN would have been re-patented 20 years ago and already be a generic drug again by now. Big Pharma would have made billions of dollars from it and millions of people suffering from the host of immune system related disorders that it helps would have gotten relief.

I personally, would never have even had to consider going to Peru to try an ayahuasca treatment, and there would have been no reason for me to write this book. Instead the progression of my disease would have halted *before* the subcortical dementia had a chance to ruin my life.

And ruin it it did.

Epilogue

One of the effects of MS that I have recently researched is that it often causes severe changes in one's personality. Changes that the person suffering from it is completely unaware of. But family and friends around the sufferer often find it very hard to tolerate.

During the course of writing this book, I so alienated my beloved wife of 25 years that we are now in the process of divorcing and she refuses to even meet with me, despite my telling her that the personality changes have been reversed.

My first son, who I helped develop into one of the most amazing, accomplished people I know, refused to communicate with me with so much as an email for over two months.

For two months even my father refused to talk to me on the telephone.

All my friends in Santa Cruz have dropped me one after another as time went by.

I find myself isolated and alone and facing having to build a completely new life for myself at the age of 54.

My one consolation is that because of LDN I actually have a chance of doing it.

One of the "side effects" of LDN is that because it triples the body's production of endorphins, one tends to see every glass as half full rather than half empty. This, I believe, is why I have been able to continue working on this book despite all the personal tragedies that have befallen me.

It's impossible to really describe what it "feels like" to lose one's cognitive abilities under MS. It's equally impossible to describe what it's like to get them back. But I know that I am one of the very few, if not the only lucky person in the world up until now that has successfully restored the damage done to his brain by MS.

When I started taking the Desoxyn, I needed 25 mg to make it through the day. After a few months I noticed I seemed to need less and less. As of a week ago, I quit taking them completely. **I am *FREE !***

My brain is clearly rewiring itself around those portions destroyed by the MS. Just as car accident victims who lose the ability to speak relearn speech in a few years, so I am relearning not only how to think again in an organized fashion, but how to function as the loving, caring person I always thought I was.

My dream is that this book will encourage those suffering as I did to take heart.

There is hope.

Don't listen to the conventional wisdom.

Don't listen to me, either.

Just Google LDN!

And find out for yourselves.

Joseph Wouk – January 13, 2009

Failure is an opportunity.
If you blame someone else,
there is no end to the blame.

Therefore the Master
fulfills his own obligations
and corrects his own mistakes.
He does what he needs to do
and demands nothing of others.

Lao Tzu

APPENDIX

This extensive appendix is designed to provide the reader with the most up to date information available on LDN and its effects on the variety of diseases that it is known to be helpful for.

Additionally, the latest clinical trials and studies are included with complete references to the scholarly or medical journals in which they were published.

This is to help the patients convince their doctors to prescribe LDN to them should they decide they want it. They should bring the book with them and show their doctors the studies relevant to their condition.

If after viewing these studies the doctor still refuses to prescribe the LDN, it might be in the patient's interest to get a second opinion from another doctor.

Table of Contents

From LDNINFO.ORG

LDN Overview

"LDN may well be the most important therapeutic breakthrough in over fifty years. It provides a new method of medical treatment by mobilizing the natural defenses of one's own immune system." — David Gluck, MD

Low Dose Naltrexone

FDA-approved naltrexone, in a low dose, can boost the immune system — helping those with HIV/AIDS, cancer, autoimmune diseases, and central nervous system disorders.

What is low-dose naltrexone and why is it important?

Low-dose naltrexone holds great promise for the millions of people worldwide with autoimmune diseases or central nervous system disorders or who face a deadly cancer.

In the developing world, LDN could provide the first low-cost, easy to administer, and side-effect-free therapy for HIV/AIDS.

Naltrexone itself was approved by the FDA in 1984 in a 50mg dose for the purpose of helping heroin or opium addicts, by blocking the effect of such drugs. By blocking opioid receptors, naltrexone also blocks the reception of the opioid hormones that our brain and adrenal glands produce: beta-endorphin and metenkephalin. Many body tissues have receptors for these endorphins and enkephalins, including virtually every cell of the body's immune system.

In 1985, Bernard Bihari, MD, a physician with a clinical practice in New York City, discovered the effects of a much smaller dose of naltrexone (approximately 3mg once a day) on the body's immune system. He found that this low dose, taken at bedtime, was able to enhance a patient's response to infection by HIV, the virus that causes AIDS. [Note: Subsequently, the optimal adult dosage of LDN has been found to be 4.5mg.]

In the mid-1990's, Dr. Bihari found that patients in his practice with cancer (such as lymphoma or pancreatic cancer) could benefit, in some cases dramatically, from LDN. In addition, people who had an autoimmune disease (such as lupus) often showed prompt control of disease activity while taking LDN.

How does LDN work?

LDN boosts the immune system by increasing the body's endorphin production, activating the body's own natural defenses.

Up to the present time, the question of "What controls the immune system?" has not been present in the curricula of medical colleges and the issue has not formed a part of the received wisdom of practicing physicians. Nonetheless, a body of research over the past two decades has pointed repeatedly to one's own endorphin secretions (our internal opioids) as playing the central role in the beneficial orchestration of the immune system, and recognition of the facts is growing.

Witness these statements from a review article of medical progress in the November 13, 2003 issue of the prestigious New England Journal of Medicine: "Opioid-Induced Immune Modulation: .... Preclinical evidence indicates overwhelmingly that opioids alter the development, differentiation, and function of immune cells, and that both innate and adaptive systems are affected.[1,2] Bone marrow progenitor cells, macrophages, natural killer cells, immature thymocytes and T cells, and B cells are all involved. The relatively recent identification of opioid-related receptors on immune cells makes it even more likely that opioids have direct effects on the immune system.[3]"

The brief blockade of opioid receptors between 2 a.m. and 4 a.m. that is caused by taking LDN at bedtime each night is believed to produce a prolonged up-regulation of vital elements of the immune system by causing an increase in endorphin and enkephalin production. Normal volunteers who have taken LDN in this fashion have been found to have much higher levels of beta-endorphins circulating in their blood in the following days. Animal research by I. Zagon, PhD, and his colleagues has shown a marked increase in metenkephalin levels as well. [Note: Additional information for Dr. Zagon can be found at the end of this page.]

Bihari says that his patients with HIV/AIDS who regularly took LDN before the availability of HAART were generally spared any deterioration of their important helper T cells (CD4+).

In human cancer, research by Zagon over many years has demonstrated inhibition of a number of different human tumors in laboratory studies by using endorphins and low dose naltrexone. It is suggested that the increased endorphin and enkephalin levels, induced by LDN, work directly on the tumors' opioid receptors — and, perhaps, induce cancer cell death (apoptosis). In addition, it is believed that they act to increase natural killer cells and other healthy immune defenses against cancer.

In general, in people with diseases that are partially or largely triggered by a deficiency of endorphins (including cancer and autoimmune diseases), or are accelerated by a deficiency of endorphins (such as HIV/AIDS), restoration of the body's normal production of endorphins is the major therapeutic action of LDN.

What diseases has it been useful for and how effective is it?

Bernard Bihari, MD, as well as other physicians and researchers, have described beneficial effects of LDN on a variety of diseases:

Cancers:

- Bladder Cancer
- Breast Cancer
- Carcinoid
- Colon & Rectal Cancer
- Glioblastoma
- Liver Cancer
- Lung Cancer (Non-Small

Other Diseases:

- ALS (Lou Gehrig's Disease)
- Alzheimer's Disease
- Ankylosing Spondylitis
- Autism Spectrum Disorders
- Behcet's Disease
- Celiac Disease
- Chronic Fatigue Syndrome

Cell)

- Lymphocytic Leukemia (chronic)

- Lymphoma (Hodgkin's and Non-Hodgkin's)

- Malignant Melanoma

- Multiple Myeloma

- Neuroblastoma

- Ovarian Cancer

- Pancreatic Cancer

- Prostate Cancer (untreated)

- Renal Cell Carcinoma

- Throat Cancer

- Uterine Cancer

- CREST syndrome

- Crohn's Disease

- Emphysema (COPD)

- Endometriosis

- Fibromyalgia

- HIV/AIDS

- Irritable Bowel Syndrome (IBS)

- Multiple Sclerosis (MS)

- Parkinson's Disease

- Pemphigoid

- Primary Lateral Sclerosis (PLS)

- Psoriasis

- Rheumatoid Arthritis

- Sarcoidosis

- Scleroderma

- Stiff Person Syndrome (SPS)

- Systemic Lupus (SLE)

- Transverse Myelitis

- Ulcerative Colitis

- Wegener's Granulomatosis

LDN has demonstrated efficacy in thousands of cases.

Cancer. As of mid-2004, Dr. Bihari reported having treated over 300 patients who had a cancer that had failed to respond to standard treatments. Of that group, some 50%, after four to six months treatment with LDN, began to demonstrate a halt in cancer growth and, of those, over one-third have shown objective signs of tumor shrinkage.

Autoimmune diseases. Within the group of patients who presented with an autoimmune disease (see above list), none have failed to respond to LDN; all have experienced a halt in progression of their illness. In many patients there was a marked remission in signs and symptoms of the disease. The greatest number of patients within the autoimmune group are people with multiple sclerosis, of whom there were some 400 in Dr. Bihari's practice. Less than 1% of these patients has ever experienced a fresh attack of MS while they maintained their regular LDN nightly therapy.

HIV/AIDS. As of September 2003, Dr. Bihari had been treating 350 AIDS patients using LDN in conjunction with accepted AIDS therapies. Over the prior 7 years over 85% of these patients showed no detectable levels of the HIV virus — a much higher success rate than most current AIDS treatments, and with no significant side effects. It is also worth noting that many HIV/AIDS patients have been living symptom-free for years taking only LDN with no other medications.

Central Nervous System disorders. Anecdotal reports continue to be received concerning beneficial effects of LDN on the course of Parkinson's disease, Alzheimer's disease, amyotrophic lateral sclerosis (ALS—Lou Gehrig's disease), and primary lateral sclerosis. Dr. Jaquelyn McCandless has found a very positive effect of LDN, in appropriately reduced dosage and applied as a transdermal cream, in children with autism.

How is it possible that one medication can impact such a wide range of disorders?

The disorders listed above all share a particular feature: in all of them, the immune system plays a central role. Low blood levels of endorphins are generally present, contributing to the disease-associated immune deficiencies.

Research by others — on neuropeptide receptors expressed by various human tumors — has found opioid receptors in many types of cancer:

- Brain tumors (both astrocytoma and glioblastoma)

- Breast cancer

- Endometrial cancer

- Head and neck squamous cell carcinoma

- Myeloid leukemia

- Lung cancer (both small cell and non-small cell)

- Neuroblastoma and others...

These findings suggest the possibility for a beneficial LDN effect in a wide variety of common cancers.

How can I obtain LDN and what will it cost?

LDN can be prescribed by your doctor, and should be prepared by a reliable compounding pharmacy.

Naltrexone is a prescription drug, so your physician would have to give you a prescription after deciding that LDN appears appropriate for you.

Naltrexone in the large 50mg size, originally manufactured by DuPont under the brand name ReVia, is now sold by Mallinckrodt as Depade and by Barr Laboratories under the generic name naltrexone.

LDN prescriptions are now being filled by hundreds of local pharmacies, as well as by some mail-order pharmacies, around the US. Some pharmacists have been grinding up the 50mg tablets of naltrexone to prepare the 4.5mg capsules of LDN; others use naltrexone, purchased as a pure powder, from a primary manufacturer.

One of the first pharmacies to do so was Irmat Pharmacy in Manhattan. Their recent price for a one-month's supply of 4.5mg LDN (30 capsules) was $38. Irmat does monthly quality control testing on its LDN, accepts prescriptions from any licensed physician, checks for insurance coverage, and includes shipment anywhere in the US or to other countries. In contrast, Gideon's Drugs charges $15 for a one month's supply of 4.5mg LDN but it does not accept insurance and it will charge for shipment.

Pharmacies that are known to be reliable compounders of LDN:

Pharmacy	Phone	Fax
Irmat Pharmacy, New York, NY	(212) 685-0500 (800) 975-2809	(212) 532-6596
Gideon's Drugs, New York, NY	(212) 575-6868	(212) 575-6334
The Compounder Pharmacy, Aurora, IL	(630) 859-0333 (800) 679-4667	(630) 859-0114
The Medicine Shoppe, Canandaigua, NY	(585) 396-9970 (800) 396-9970	(585) 396-7264
Skip's Pharmacy, Boca Raton, FL	(561) 218-0111 (800) 553-7429	(561) 218-8873
Smith's Pharmacy, Toronto, Canada	(416) 488-2600 (800) 361-6624	(416) 484-8855
Dickson Chemist, Glasgow, Scotland	+44-141-647-8032 +44-800-027-0673	+44-141-647-8032

IMPORTANT: Make sure to specify that you do NOT want LDN in a slow-release form.

Reports have been received from patients that their pharmacies have been supplying a *slow-release form* of naltrexone. Pharmacies should be instructed NOT to provide LDN in an "SR" or slow-release or timed-release form. Unless the low dose of naltrexone is in an unaltered form, which permits it to reach a prompt "spike" in the blood stream, its therapeutic effects may be inhibited.

Fillers. Capsules of LDN necessarily contain a substantial percentage of neutral inactive filler. Experiments by the compounding pharmacist, Dr. Skip Lenz, have demonstrated that the use of calcium carbonate as a filler will interfere with absorption of the LDN capsule. Therefore, it is suggested that calcium carbonate filler not be employed in compounding LDN capsules. He recommends either Avicel, lactose (if lactose intolerance is not a problem), or sucrose fillers as useful fast-release fillers.

IMPORTANT: Make sure to fill your Rx at a compounding pharmacy that has a reputation for consistent reliability in the quality of the LDN it delivers.

The FDA has found a significant error rate in compounded prescriptions produced at randomly selected pharmacies. Dr. Bihari has reported seeing adverse effects from this problem. Please see our report, Reliability Problem With Compounding Pharmacies. Please see the above list of recommended pharmacies for some suggested sources.

What dosage and frequency should my physician prescribe?

The usual adult dosage is 4.5mg taken once daily at night. Because of the rhythms of the body's production of master hormones, LDN is best taken between 9pm and 3am. Most patients take it at bedtime.

Notable exceptions:

- People who have multiple sclerosis that has led to muscle spasms are advised to use only 3mg daily and to maintain that dosage.

- For intial dosage of LDN in those patients who have Hashimoto's thyroiditis with hypothyroidism and who are taking thyroid hormone replacement medication, please read Cautionary Warnings, below.

Rarely, the naltrexone may need to be purchased as a solution — in distilled water — with 1mg per ml dispensed with a 5ml medicine dropper. If LDN is used in a liquid form, it is important to keep it refrigerated.

The therapeutic dosage range for LDN is from 1.75mg to 4.5mg every night. Dosages below this range are likely to have no effect at all, and dosages above this range are likely to block endorphins for too long a period of time and interfere with its effectiveness.

IMPORTANT: Make sure to specify that you do NOT want LDN in a slow-release form (see above).

Are there any side effects or cautionary warnings?

Side effects:

LDN has virtually no side effects. Occasionally, during the first week's use of LDN, patients may complain of some difficulty sleeping. This rarely persists after the first week. Should it do so, dosage can be reduced from 4.5mg to 3mg nightly.

Cautionary warnings:

1. Because LDN blocks opioid receptors throughout the body for three or four hours, people using medicine that is an opioid agonist, i.e. narcotic medication — such as Ultram (tramadol), morphine, Percocet, Duragesic patch or codeine-containing medication — should not take LDN until such medicine is completely out of one's system. Patients who have become dependant on daily use of narcotic-containing pain medication may require 10 days to 2 weeks of slowly weaning off of such drugs entirely (while first substituting full doses of non-narcotic pain medications) before being able to begin LDN safely.

2. Those patients who are taking thyroid hormone replacement for a diagnosis of Hashimoto's thyroiditis with *hypo*thyroidism ought to begin LDN at the lowest range (1.5mg for an adult). Be aware that LDN may lead to a prompt decrease in the autoimmune disorder, which then may require a rapid reduction in the dose of thyroid hormone replacement in order to avoid symptoms of *hyper*thyroidism.

3. Full-dose naltrexone (50mg) carries a cautionary warning against its use in those with liver disease. This warning was placed because of adverse liver effects that were found in experiments involving 300mg daily. The 50mg dose does not apparently produce impairment of liver function nor, of course, do the much smaller 3mg and 4.5mg doses.

4. People who have received organ transplants and who therefore are taking immunosuppressive medication on a permanent basis are cautioned against the use of LDN because it may act to counter the effect of those medications.

When will the low-dose use of naltrexone become FDA approved?

Although naltrexone itself is an FDA-approved drug, the varied uses of LDN still await application to the FDA after related scientific clinical trials.

The FDA approved naltrexone at the 50mg dosage in 1984. LDN (in the 3mg or 4.5mg dosage) has not yet been submitted for approval because the prospective clinical trials that are required for FDA approval need to be funded at the cost of many millions of dollars.

The successful results of the first US medical center research on LDN, an open-label trial that tested the use of LDN in Crohn's disease (details here), was presented in May 2006 by Professor Jill Smith of the Pennsylvania State University College of Medicine. The National Institutes of Health has granted $500,000 for Dr. Smith's group to continue the study as a larger placebo-controlled scientific trial of LDN in Crohn's disease.

All physicians understand that appropriate off-label use of an already FDA-approved medication such as naltrexone is perfectly ethical and legal. Because naltrexone itself has already passed animal toxicity studies, one could expect that once testing is able to begin, LDN could complete its clinical trials in humans and receive FDA approval for one or more uses within two to four years.

What You Can Do

Talk to your doctor.

If you are suffering from HIV/AIDS, cancer, or an autoimmune disease, LDN could help. In AIDS and cancer therapy, LDN is often used in conjunction with other medications.

Cancer. Anyone with cancer or a pre-cancerous condition should consider LDN. Many use LDN as a preventive treatment. Post-treatment, others have been using LDN to prevent a recurrence of their cancer. LDN has been shown in many cases to work with virtually incurable cancers such as neuroblastoma, multiple myeloma, and pancreatic cancer.

HIV/AIDS. As an AIDS drug, LDN leads to far fewer side effects than the standard "AIDS cocktail." When used in conjunction with HAART therapies, LDN can boost T-cell populations, prevent disfiguring lipodystrophy, and lower rates of treatment failure.

Do not be afraid to approach your doctors — physicians today are increasingly open to learning about new therapies in development. Tell your doctors about this website, or print out and hand them the information, and let them weigh the evidence.

Tell others.

If someone you know has HIV/AIDS, cancer, an autoimmune disease, or one of the aforementioned central nervous system disorders, LDN could save them from a great deal of suffering. If they use e-mail, send them the address of this website (www.lowdosenaltrexone.org). Or, print out the site and mail them the information.

Help spread the word to the media, the medical community, and to developing countries.

Low-dose naltrexone has the potential to reduce the terrible human loss now taking place throughout the globe. It is a drug that could prevent millions of children from becoming AIDS orphans. It is a drug that could be a powerful ally in the war against cancer.

If you or someone you know has connections in the media, the medical community, or to those in developing countries involved in AIDS policy or treatment, please let them know about LDN.

Additional Information

- **Bernard Bihari, MD**, is the discoverer of the major clinical effects of low dose naltrexone. A private practitioner in Manhattan, he retired in March 2007. Dr. Bihari is a Board-certified specialist in Psychiatry and Neurology. Dr. Bihari's curriculum vitae.

- **David Gluck, MD**, is the editor of this website, *ldninfo.org*. He is a Board-certified specialist in both Internal Medicine and Preventive Medicine. Dr. Gluck has served as medical director for JCPenney and MetLife, and is now semi-retired, living and working in New York City.

- **Ian S. Zagon, PhD**, has spent over two decades in doing basic research concerning endorphins. He is Professor of Neural and Behavioral Sciences, Pennsylvania State University, Dept. of Neural and Behavioral Sciences, H-109, Hershey Medical Center, Hershey, PA 17033; office phone: (717) 531-6409; email: isz1@psu.edu; website.

Footnotes

1. Roy S, Loh HH. *Effects of opioids on the immune system.* Neurochem Res 1996;21:1375-1386

2. Risdahl JM, Khanna KV, Peterson PK, Molitor TW. *Opiates and infection.* J Neuroimmunol 1998;83:4-18

3. Makman MH. *Morphine receptors in immunocytes and neurons.* Adv Neuroimmunol 1994;4:69-82

How LDN works and was discovered - Interview with Dr. Bihari

Dr. Kamau B. Kokayi Interviews Dr. Bihari
September 23, 2003
WBAI in New York City

"Global Medicine Review"

Dr. Bihari: Well, we were treating heroin addicts, and in 1984 a new drug for the treatment of addiction came out. It was called Naltrexone, and it was designed to block the heroin "high"and it was a flop. I used it for a lot of patients, as did most addiction doctors across the country. At 50 milligrams a day, it made people feel terrible. Not that it blocked the heroin so much as it blocked their own endorphins, which is a source of our sense of well-being, so that people couldn't sleep.

Dr. Kokayi: Your own opium, basically.

Dr. Bihari: Right. Your own equivalent. That's what heroin is. And I knew from work that had been done by the National Institute on Drug Abuse in developing the drug that it had the ability to trigger the body into making more endorphins, but at the high 50 milligram dosage, the dose was too high. It blocks those endorphins. About six months later our addicts began dying in large numbers of AIDS. I ran HIV tests on about a hundred addicts, and fifty percent were already HIV positive. This was in 1985; currently it's eighty eighty-five percent around the country. And we began looking for some way to approach this new disease, with a view to the idea that this disease was likely to turn into a worldwide epidemic.

Dr. Kokayi: That was about the time where people were just being blasted with AZT with horrific results.

Dr. Bihari: Right. There was nothing else available. When I discovered that people with HIV had less than twenty percent of the normal levels of endorphins, that meant that the virus not only kills the immune system cells, it also weakens the whole immune system, so that it's not as able to fight the virus. We began looking for ways to use this drug to raise endorphins without blocking them. We hired a laboratory scientist to measure endorphin levels.

We'd measure in the afternoon, then we'd give the first dose at bedtime that night. Then we'd measure again at the same time the next day; then again at one week, and again at one month. We found that doses in the range of 1.75 to 4.5 milligrams (which is just a fraction of the recommended dosage to addicts) would trigger or jumpstart endorphin production during the night. Except with exercise, endorphins are made only between two and four in the morning. The brain sends a message out to the adrenal and pituitary glands and tells them to make endorphins. Giving a dose three, four, five hours before that, at bedtime, is enough to make that message from the brain much stronger.

Dr. Kokayi: Were you able to document that the levels of endorphins were then actually raised?

Dr. Bihari: The level of endorphins went up by two hundred to three hundred percent. We then started a little foundation and did a placebo-controlled trial in which half the patients got the drug and half got sugar pills. A year later when we broke the code, we discovered that people with HIV who took the drug had only an eight percent death rate in the year, while people who were on the placebo had a thirty-three percent death rate. And of course they had many more infections and their immune system declined. That was a startling discovery.

Dr. Kokayi: Now let me jump ahead, because I'm always curious about why this therapy hasn't gotten the kind of publicity specifically for this disease.

Dr. Bihari: Well, at that time there was very little treatment. AZT came out about ' 87, and as you mentioned, it was not only a flop but made some people sicker. At the time we did the study, there was nothing available. So I met with doctors in New York and in San Francisco (where the largest number of HIV doctors were at that time) and described this drug and how it worked, and about forty to fifty doctors on the east and west coast began using it. Unfortunately, they measured effectiveness by whether or not the numbers of the immune system cells that are crucial in AIDS -- the CD4 cells -- were rising. On this drug, CD4 cells don't rise in people with AIDS. As I knew from the study, and have known since, they simply stop dropping. That means you can freeze the disease wherever it is. And if somebody is only mildly immune-suppressed, they stay that way.

Dr. Kokayi: That's so important…

Dr. Bihari: It stops progression. It stops the count from growing. I have patients going back as much as seventeen years who haven't lost an immune system cell in that time. They're very healthy.

Dr. Kokayi: Wow, that needs to be on the evening news.

Dr. Bihari: The trouble was, we wrote a paper, but couldn't get it published. Nobody understood the concept.

Dr. Kokayi: You're using the dose homeopathically. You're using it not for the effect that the medicine has on the person, but for the body's reaction to the medicine.

Dr. Bihari: It strengthens the body's own defenses. Rather than directly attacking, the way antibiotics attack bacteria, or the way chemotherapy tries to attack cancer cells, or the way anti-viral drugs attack viruses, the purpose of this is to take a weak defense (which people with AIDS or cancer have), and strengthen it so that the body can fight the disease more effectively.

Dr. Kokayi: I've often made the point that therapies like acupuncture, therapies that are foreign to the cultural mindset of doctors and the American public, these therapies can be effective, but they won't be included or in mainstream medicine because the concept is so foreign.

Dr. Bihari: It's a different model of understanding the body -- how it works and how disease works. I think eventually there will be changes in the paradigm of the way we think about diseases, and it's going to be a struggle. But I think oncologists in particular are getting more and more frustrated with the failure of chemotherapy.

Dr. Kokayi: Well, about time.

Dr. Bihari: The people I talk to at the National Cancer Institute, and the Food and Drug Administration, are very negative. All they get from drug companies are proposals to test new, more toxic chemotherapies, and they're really looking very hard for non-toxic ways of modifying the behavior of the cancer cells so that they stop the cancer from growing.

Dr. Kokayi: Over the years have you had to modify what you were actually doing with Naltrexone? Or is the initial model impetus pretty much on point?

Dr. Bihari: The initial model was pretty much on point. A small dose at bedtime increases endorphin production during the night. In somebody who has a disease which is related to low endorphins, the endorphins go back up to normal by the next day. … [station break] ….

Dr. Kokayi: … can you tell us about some of the work with Naltrexone and cancer?

Dr. Bihari: During that year, when we were doing our first AIDS trial, an old friend of mine called. Five years earlier, she'd had Non-Hodgkin's Lymphoma. It had initially responded to chemotherapy, but it had grown back after her husband died. Her oncologist refused to treat her, saying it would be resistant to chemo the second time. She knew what I'd been doing, and she called me and said, "Bernie, do you think your AIDS drug would help my cancer?" So I dug around and I found a large body of literature showing that when you give endorphins, metenkephalins, beta endorphins and even low dose Naltrexone to mice that had human cancer transplanted, that there is about an 80 percent recovery rate. I gave her the drug in the same dose we were using in the AIDS trial. She had large masses in her groin, her neck, her chest, and her abdomen, and they all slowly shrank and disappeared over a (inaudible) period. (Inaudible) taking the drug every night.

Dr. Kokayi: Wow! You know, even if that's just an anecdote….

Dr. Bihari: Yes.

Dr. Kokay: I mean, everyone who has that disease deserves a chance to see if they're going to be an anecdote as well.

Dr. Bihari: It was actually her idea. She stayed on the drug, and died about eight years later, in her late seventies, of her third heart attack, which was unrelated. Then I was in Paris the following summer, presenting a paper at an AIDS conference, and I met a woman who had a cancer called malignant melanoma. It starts in the skin, and in her case it had spread to the brain. She had four large brain tumors. The oncologist told her family that she had perhaps three months to live. When I got back to New York, I shipped her the drug from a pharmacy that was making it for our study. She started on it, and her neurological symptoms from the tumors in her brain slowly disappeared.

Seven or eight months later she went back to the oncologist, had a cat scan of the brain done, and the tumors were gone.

Dr. Kokayi: Fantastic.

Dr. Bihari: That was eighteen years ago, and she stayed on it.

Dr. Kokayi: This is such a non-toxic, simple [inaudible].

Dr. Bihari: There are absolutely no side effects. I continued doing a lot of the AIDS work, but the last four or five years I've gotten much more interested in other uses. We stumbled on the fact, also by chance, that the drug works very well for almost all, if not all, of the autoimmune diseases like multiple sclerosis, rheumatoid arthritis, lupus, sarcoidosis, and --

Dr. Kokayi: When you say "it works", what actually happens? What's been your experience?

Dr. Bihari: Well, what happens is that the disease activity stops, as long as people stay on it. If they have damage to the brain and spinal cord with multiple sclerosis, that doesn't disappear, because that's due to scarring, but they stop getting new attacks. I've had people on Low Dose Naltrexone for years. The longest is a friend of my daughter, who's been on it for eighteen years and has not had an attack as long as she stayed on it.

Dr. Kokayi: So it's almost as if it's up-regulating the endorphin production but somehow the endorphins actually block or inhibit the effect of the antibodies from attacking the tissue.

Dr. Bihari: Not directly. It's more that the autoimmune diseases are beginning to look more and more like they're diseases of endorphin deficiency. [Inaudible] models of all the diseases I mention that can be bred in mice, the endorphin levels are always fifteen to twenty percent of normal compared with normal mice. [Female Voice] How can you naturally increase endorphin levels?

Dr. Bihari: There's only three or four ways that I know. First, Naltrexone increases them substantially, two to three hundred percent in people with low levels. Second, aerobic exercise increases them, but not as much. If you do an hour of exercise four or five times a week it will last three, four hours, and that's one of the reasons that exercise helps prevent cancer. A third way, oddly, is acupuncture. Acupuncture, especially when used in treating addicts, increases endorphin levels in the blood and the spinal fluid. And chocolate increases it.

Dr. Kokayi: [Inaudible] will be glad to hear that. Female Voice: [inaudible] It actually works out, because you're going to eat your chocolate and then run to the gym.

Dr. Bihari: Chocolate has a substance in it called Phenylalanine, which slows endorphins from being broken down in the body.

Dr. Kokayi: And that's basically an amino acid that we find….

Dr. Bihari: Yes, that's the food that has it in the largest amount. And only people with a rare disease called [inaudible] can't eat chocolate.

Dr. Kokayi: So some people will run to the health food store and get Phenylalanine.

Dr. Bihari: Well, Phenylalanine is helpful if you're raising your endorphins by other means. Then it keeps them from decaying. They last much longer. But the crucial thing still seems to me to be the Naltrexone. Over the last five or six years, I've treated about 420 patients who have various kinds of cancer with low dose Naltrexone. Occasionally, for people who come to me with very advanced cancer, I add intravenous metenkephalin, which is an endorphin... intravenously, three times a week. It improved immune function substantially, and had no side effects, but that's generally not needed. Among the people I've treated with Naltrexone for various kinds of cancer, on the average the cancer stops growing in about two-thirds. For half of that group, it eventually -- after six, seven, eight months -- goes on to slowly shrink and disappear.

Dr. Kokayi: And that's about forty percent.

Dr. Bihari: Higher.

Dr. Kokayi: Well, it's about forty percent of the total number.

Dr. Bihari: Sixty-five percent actually benefit and don't go on to develop [inaudible]. Thirty percent go into remission.

Dr. Kokayi: That's phenomenal. I don't think there's any chemo or radiating oncologist with numbers like that.

Dr. Bihari: There's no downside. One of the reasons that the war on cancer failed is that the oncologists doing the research failed to take into account that chemotherapy really wipes out the immune system, which the body needs to fight cancer cells. So they are giving drugs that kill cancer cells, but at the same time weakening the body's defense against cancer. Naltrexone strengthens the body's defense, and the increased endorphins kill cancer cells directly. Also, the immune system when it's strengthened kills cancer cells through its natural killer cells.

Dr. Kokayi: What you're saying is, that a boost in endorphin levels also activates other components of the immune system.

Dr. Bihari: The endorphins are the hormones centrally involved in regulating the immune system. About 95% of the regulation or orchestration comes from endorphins. People with cancer -- especially adults – have very low natural killer cells. They have a weakened immune system. I've discovered, after seeing such a large number of people, that the vast majority of them have experienced major life stresses lasting weeks, months to years – anywhere from two to six years before they get the cancer.

Dr. Kokayi: That was one of my other questions. What really can keep those endorphin levels down in the body?

Dr. Bihari: If a child gets sick -- children are supposed to outlive us -- so if a child gets sick and dies, or if you have a very bad marital break-up, or if you discover a business partner is embezzling money and it takes a couple of years to straighten out... If you wake up every morning under stress -- really serious stress, not everyday stress -- really serious stress, this can lower your endorphin production, and it never returns to normal. So the person then walks around with low endorphins. The body makes cancer cells all the time, but usually the immune system kills them as they are forming. But if your endorphin levels are low, then your immune system is weak, the cancers grow and you become much more vulnerable. The same thing with exposure to really toxic substances.

Dr. Kokayi: Right. I'm wondering, I'm sure the listening audience would like to get an idea. If you could just run down a list of some of the cancers that you have successfully treated, types of cancers that have seemed to respond where the opiate levels play a prominent role.

Dr. Bihari: Well, first one of the things we discovered was that almost all cancers have a lot of receptors for endorphins on the cell surface, and that seems to be necessary for it to work. Some of the cancers that respond most dramatically are Multiple Myeloma, Lymphoma, Hodgkin's disease, breast cancer, all the cancers of the gastrointestinal tract, like pancreatic cancer, non small-cell cancer of the lung, the kind associated with smoking. I've got several patients with tumors that have stopped growing; they have no symptoms, and then after a year, year and a half, in about half of that group, the tumors start shrinking and disappear.

Dr. Kokayi: This is lung cancer?

Dr. Bihari: These are lung cancers due to smoking.

Dr. Kokayi: Because there's really --

Dr. Bihari: Very common.

Dr. Kokayi: It's very common, but therapeutic effectiveness --

Dr. Bihari: There's nothing --

Dr. Kokayi: There's nothing, right --

Dr. Bihari: My own attitude about chemotherapy in patients I see with cancer, is if they have one of those rare cancers that's very sensitive to chemotherapy, like cancer of the testicle, I encourage them to do that, to take it, and take Naltrexone afterwards to prevent recurrence. These drugs are licensed to treat cancer. Naltrexone is not yet licensed to treat cancer, although it's a licensed drug. It's been on the market for nineteen years. It's use in these low doses is called an "off-label" use. Any doctor can prescribe it. And growing numbers of oncologists and neurologists in the country are prescribing it.

Dr. Kokayi: I think it would be interesting you know just to talk a little bit about the process … a lot of physicians don't really know about it and it's not talked about. This is a big deal.

Dr. Bihari: Well, I think it could turn out to be a big deal when it's picked up, if it's picked up. We set up a web site, www.ldninfo.org, which brings up about thirty pages of written material describing all the diseases, and how they respond, and how many cases we have of them. There's some small trials going on, there's two trials in people with Crohn's Disease, which is an autoimmune disease of the small intestine, one in Jerusalem, and one in New York. There's a trial in Israel for multiple sclerosis. The national cancer institute has copies of twenty charts of my patients who have agreed to share their charts. These are people who have done well on Naltrexone when nothing else could explain how well they've done. They intend to present them to a committee for recommendations as to whether to invest and test it in the network of cancer research.

Dr. Kokayi: You know, when I think about Africa and AIDS, this is exactly the kind of medicine there needs to be there….

Dr. Bihari: This is perfect. In fact, we've been working with the largest pharmaceutical company in the developing world called (inaudible) in India to get a trial going, probably in Africa, in the Republic of South Africa, in which half the HIV patients get the drug, half get a placebo, and they should be able to show in about nine months, using two to three hundred patients, that this drug stops progression. Once it does, it will be manufacturable at less than ten dollars per year per person. That's been the big problem -- the anti-HIV drugs are so expensive. The average income in Africa is about eighty dollars per year.

Dr. Kokayi: I can only imagine just the financial stress that you've had to go through just to keep this whole project alive. It's one thing to prescribe things as an individual doctor, but to get recognition within the scientific community is a bit difficult.

Dr. Bihari: It really bothers me when doctors say, "Oh, I can't prescribe that, because he hasn't done a placebo-controlled trial." That's a full-time job, for two, three years involving eight or nine centers around the country. I'm working with a number of diseases in my office, and a lot of money goes out paying for the website, for patents to cover low dose naltexone, and (inaudible) things like that. It's very veryexpensive. But I can't stop doing it. My wife and I would love to do some traveling -- I think we've earned it -- but I really can't stop until the drug is out there. It's as much of a burden as it does a pleasure.

Dr. Kokayi: I really hope that at least your sharing with our listening audience today helps to make people more aware. People should be clamoring for it. We're running out of time, but I wanted to go back to the treatment of autoimmune diseases. I always pictured them as the body is attacking its own tissues. I pictured these antibodies actually honing in there. But you're saying that, in large measure it's an actual endorphin deficiency.

Dr. Bihari: It's an endorphin deficiency which weakens the immune system, so that certain cells in the body forget to distinguish between the body tissues and bacteria or viruses, so when these cells are activated by an infection they attack the bacteria and they attack you. Restoring the immune function to normal stops that. So far, the drug works dramatically in all the diseases that are labeled autoimmune diseases.

Dr. Kokayi: And you've treated lupus with this.

Dr. Bihari: I've treated -- I have two dozen cases of lupus. I have about the same number of people with rheumatoid arthritis. I have about twenty people with Crohn's Disease. A number of rheumatologists who specialize in these diseases in New York are now beginning to use it, because we have cases in common, and they see.

Dr. Kokayi: Right

Dr. Bihari: Because they're using cancer drugs Female Voice:

Dr. Bihari, is this being used with children with ADD?

Dr. Bihari: I doubt that it would work, knowing the nature of ADD. I doubt that it would work. It doesn't do everything for everybody. I don't think it would.

Dr. Kokayi: Again, going back to the idea of giving a medicine that at a higher dose actually blocks the chemical system, but a lower dose actually augments it.

Dr. Bihari: And enhances the body's defenses -- that's essential.

Dr. Koyayi: This idea gives the pharmaceutical industry something to do, rather than giving people high doses of medication.

Dr. Bihari: It certainly would. It will take this drug to be licensed, picked up by a pharmaceutical company and tested, licensed, and once it's widely used, then this approach to medicine -- every medical researcher will start thinking about it. It's an entirely different approach to the body and illness.

Dr. Kokayi: What is the next step? Is there anything that the listening audience can do that might be helpful for to make this more -- not even make it more available, because it's just a prescription any doctor can write. I guess it's the information --

Dr. Bihari: The information, getting it from the website, getting doctors to prescribe it. I'm always happy to take calls from doctors and spend as much time as I need, because the more doctors prescribe it, the more widely used it will be. Currently, as far as we can calculate it, over eighty thousand people in the U.S. and western Europe are on the drug, and the numbers are increasing rapidly. From: http://www.gazorpa.com/interview.html

LDN and Multiple Sclerosis

Frequently Asked Questions

What is Low Dose Naltrexone?

Naltrexone is short for Naltrexone Hydrochloride (C20H23NO4-HCl), an opiate antagonist. Naltrexone was approved by the FDA (at a 50mg dosage) in 1984 for opiate addiction, and again in 1995 for alcohol abuse. At a much lower dose (1.75-4.5mg), it has been gaining popularity as a treatment for symptoms of auto-immune disorders such as Multiple Sclerosis. Low Dose Naltrexone is administered orally, usually in capsule form.

What MS symptoms does LDN help?

Primarily neuromuscular spasm, fatigue, and urinary problems, although patients have also reported improvements of other symptoms. In addition, patients who start LDN while in the middle of an acute relapse often show rapid resolution of the attack.

Does LDN halt progression of MS?

Evidence suggests that LDN can significantly reduce the chances of either a relapse or progression for many MS patients.

How does LDN work?

It is believed that LDN briefly obstructs the effects of brain endorphins (the brain's natural painkillers). Sensing an endorphin deficit, the pituitary signals for increased production of endorphins, which re-balances the immune system, thus reducing the activity of the MS. The effect lasts around 18 hours.

But how can this work? Isn't MS is caused by an overactive immune system? Although there is a long-held theory that MS might be caused by an overactive immune system, this theory has never been proven. Recent clinical studies indicate that this theory might not be true at all. The October 2004 issue of The Archives of Neurology reports a clinical study which found that intravenous immunoglobulin therapy applied after the first signs of MS significantly reduced the probability of developing clinically definite multiple sclerosis. Patients receiving this immune-system boosting therapy also suffered fewer brain lesions. [Intravenous Immunoglobulin Treatment Following the First Demyelinating Event Suggestive of Multiple Sclerosis; a

Randomized Double Blind, Placebo-Controlled Trial; Arch. Neurol. Oct. 2004; 61:1515-1520.]

How fast does LDN work?

Although some patients have no symptom changes, around two-thirds of MS patients report some symptom improvement within the first few days. Other patients report improvement over the course of several weeks or even months.

What dosage and frequency are usually prescribed?

The usual adult dosage of LDN for the treatment of MS is 1.75-4.5mg taken orally once daily at bedtime. Because of the natural rhythms of the body's hormone production, LDN is best taken between 9pm and 2am. It is generally recommended that the patient begin on 3.0mg per day, and adjust the dosage if necessary. Prescribing 1.5mg capsules allows easy adjustment of dosage. (For example, the patient can take either 2 capsules for 3mg, or 3 capsules for a 4.5mg dose.)

How is LDN prepared?

LDN is usually prepared by a compounding pharmacist, who makes capsules by either grinding up 50mg Naltrexone tablets, or using Naltrexone powder purchased from a primary manufacturer. (The most popular Naltrexone tablet is the 50mg "ReVia" Naltrexone tablet, usually prescribed for treatment of drug and alcohol addictions.)

LDN may also be prepared in a solution of distilled water, with 1mg per ml dispensed with a 5ml medicine dropper. If LDN is used in a liquid form, it is recommended that it be refrigerated.

Are there any side effects?

All sources indicate that LDN has virtually no side effects. Some patients report vivid dreams, and occasionally, during the first week of use, patients may complain of difficulty sleeping. (Reports indicate that sleep disturbance is rare, occurring in less than 2% of users.) If this persists after the first week, dosage can be reduced from 4.5mg to 3mg. Full-dose Naltrexone (50mg 3x day) carries a cautionary warning for patients with liver disease. (This warning was placed because adverse liver effects were noted in early experiments involving 300mg daily, given for alcohol abuse.) The 50mg dose does not apparently produce impairment of liver function nor, of course, does the much smaller 3mg - 4.5mg dose.

LDN is virtually non-toxic, simple to administer, and, compared with other MS drug therapy, very inexpensive – usually costing less than $40 per month.

What about cautionary warnings?

Because LDN blocks opioid receptors throughout the body for three or four hours, people using narcotic medication such as Ultram, morphine, Percocet, Tramadol, Duragesic patch or codeine should not take LDN until such medicine is completely out of the system. Steroids would counteract the effects of LDN, and so should not be combined. LDN should probably not be taken during pregnancy.

LDN should not be used by people already receiving interferon (Beta Seron, Avonex, or Rebif). Because LDN stimulates the immune system and interferon suppresses it, the two therapies are incompatible. The combination of these therapies does not cause any adverse reactions, but it is believed that they cancel out each other's effectiveness.

What does it feel like to be on LDN?

At both high and low dosages, patients taking Naltrexone usually say they are largely unaware of being on medication. Naltrexone usually has no psychological effects and patients (at both high and low dosages) don't feel either "high" or "down" while they are on naltrexone. It is not addicting.

Why isn't LDN routinely prescribed for MS?

Many physicians simply have not yet learned about the positive effects of LDN on MS symptoms. Because Naltrexone is a generic medication, there are no commercial marketing campaigns to increase awareness of LDN in the medical community. Other doctors may be hesitant to prescribe LDN because it hasn't yet been approved as an MS treatment by the FDA.

Why hasn't LDN been approved by the FDA for MS?

Naltrexone (in the higher 50mg dosage) was approved by the FDA in 1984 for opiate abuse therapy, and again in 1995 for alcohol addiction. Its safety and efficacy have been proven in clinical trials. In the much lower dosage of 3 or 4.5mg, Naltrexone has not yet been submitted for FDA approval. Federal regulations prevent the FDA from approving LDN as an MS therapy until it undergoes specific clinical trials for MS.

Why hasn't LDN gone through a clinical trial as an MS therapy?

Clinical trials are usually initiated and funded by pharmaceutical companies, and these companies are not interested in promoting or marketing LDN.

Why aren't pharmaceutical companies interested in exploring the possibility of LDN as an MS therapy? Naltrexone was developed so long ago, it is now a generic drug, manufactured by many different companies. Since no single company owns exclusive manufacturing rights, Naltrexone can be manufactured and sold very inexpensively by any pharmaceutical company.

This means that LDN can't make anyone any money. Pharmaceutical companies are not eager to fund clinical trials for a drug that will make them no profit. Also, if LDN were FDA-approved and became a preferred treatment for MS, the pharmaceutical companies who make the expensive ABCR drugs could lose millions of dollars.

Are there any plans for a clinical trial for LDN as an MS therapy?

In May 2007, the MindBrain Consortium, the Department of Psychiatry of Summa Hospital System of Akron, Ohio, and the Oak Clinic for the treatment of Multiple Sclerosis, announced a study of the effects of treating MS with LDN.

In March 2007, the University of California, San Francisco Medical Center, implemented a double-blind, randomized, placebo-controlled, crossover-design study of the effects of LDN on 80 MS patents.

In December 2006, a study of LDN in MS was begun in Milan by neurological researcher, Dr. Maira Gironi.

In August 2004, the LDN Research Trust (www.ldnresearchtrust.org) was created in England. Organized by a group of patients who have been helped by LDN, the Trust's mission is to raise funds for the initiation of clinical trials for LDN. In conjunction with the Trust, Dr Alasdair Coles, a neurologist and MS specialist from Cambridge University, and Dr Robert Lawrence of Wales, himself an MS patient, are currently working on a proposal for a clinical trial of LDN for the treatment of MS.

Since LDN has also shown promise as a therapy for other autoimmune disorders, there has research activity in that area. In September 2007, the Institutional Review Board in Bamako, Mali, approved plans for a clinical trial of LDN in HIV-infected citizens of Mali. In July 2007, Stanford Systems Neuroscience and Pain Lab began organizing a study of LDN for the treatment of fibromyalgia.

Has LDN as an MS therapy been reported in any of the major medical journals?

Most medical journals are not interested in reviewing a drug therapy that has not yet had a clinical trial. However, the peer-reviewed medical journal Medical Hypothesis recently published an article about the LDN's success as an MS therapy.

(For full text, see: ldners. org/Articles/LDN_Medical_Hypotheses.pdf)

Can a doctor legally prescribe LDN?

Yes. While it is illegal for a pharmaceutical company to market or promote a drug for a use other than that approved by the FDA, it is NOT illegal for a physician to prescribe an FDA-approved drug for a non-FDA-approved use. This is called an "off-label" prescription, and physicians do it all the time. (Neurontin, for example, was approved by the FDA in 1993 for the treatment of epilepsy; yet it is routinely prescribed off-label for the treatment of MS.) All physicians understand that the responsible off-label use of an FDA-approved medication such as Naltrexone is perfectly ethical and legal.

Who first thought of using Low Dose Naltrexone for MS?

Initial research on LDN was conducted by Ian S. Zagon, Ph.D., Professor of Neural and Behavioral Sciences at Pennsylvania State University. The use of LDN for MS is credited to Dr. Bernard Bihari, a practicing neurologist in New York. Dr. Bihari, who received his MD from Harvard and is board-certified in psychiatry and neurology, began prescribing LDN for his MS patients in 1985.

Does anyone profit from the promotion and sale of LDN?

No. Some people are initially suspicious of LDN, thinking that it might be an internet "snake-oil" scheme, but no one markets or sells LDN for profit. Naltrexone is an inexpensive, generic medication, manufactured by a number of large pharmaceutical corporations. Low-Dose Naltrexone is compounded at individual compounding pharmacies, and is not marketed by anyone.

How many MS patients are taking LDN for Multiple Sclerosis?

No one is sure of the exact number, but it is known that thousands of MS patients worldwide are now using LDN, and the number is increasing. Without the financial support of the pharmaceutical industry, the growing reputation of LDN has been driven solely by positive reports from MS patients.

Are MS patients getting positive results from LDN?

A review of the anecdotal evidence shows that most MS patients taking LDN have experienced considerable improvement, often within days or weeks of beginning the treatment.

Pharmaceutical Information about Low Dose Naltrexone

The protocol is 1.5 to 4.5mg at bedtime. It must not be a timed-release preparation and should
be given at bedtime. Up until recently, Dr. Bihari had routinely used 3 mg, reducing it down to as low
as 1.5 mg in the rare patient who experienced a mild sleep disturbance. (Many patients report
improved sleeping.) However, recently, he has noted that some patients who did not respond to 3
mg did respond to 4.5mg and has begun to use this dose more frequently. No more than 4.5mg
must be used. Occasionally, lower doses are necessary.

The usual, commercial oral preparation of naltrexone is 50 mg; so, the 1.5 to 4.5 mg dose must be
made up by a compounding pharmacy. A month's supply should run about $30. Although there are
no known significant side effects to the treatment, in about 1 out of 50 patients, the patient will
experience a sleep disturbance. In this case, Dr. Bihari recommends that the pharmacy make up a
100-ml. solution containing naltrexone in distilled water at a concentration of 1 mg/ml. The patient is
told to take 1 to 1 ½ ml. at bedtime—possibly working up to 2 ml. or 2 mg.

--- Michael B. Schachter, M.D., CNS, F.A.C.A.
December 6, 2001

From LDNINFO.ORG

LDN and HIV/AIDS

In Brief

Since the mid-1980's, low dose naltrexone (LDN) has consistently demonstrated a markedly beneficial effect in the treatment of HIV/AIDS. There are a score of such patients who, even today, continue to successfully use only LDN. When combined with HAART, LDN has shown itself to be an absolute preventive for lipodystrophy, as well as a synergistic therapy that diminishes viral breakthroughs and bolsters the restoration of CD4 cell levels.

Recent Developments

> Treating HIV Using LDN Alone

Dr. Bihari reports that, as of November 2001, a group of 18 such patients had an average of 9.5 years of known HIV-positive status. They had been taking LDN continuously for an average of almost 7 years, and none had participated in regular maintenance therapy with HAART. Had these patients been untreated, their CD4 counts by now should have been at quite low levels and their clinical status should have been perilous.

Instead, the most recent laboratory data for these patients shows that the vital indicators of immune status have, on average, declined only minimally during the many years. The average CD4 count within the group is 445 cells (normal = 550-1500) and the average CD4% is 28.6% (normal = 27%-53%). And, indeed, they all remain free of opportunistic infections and other indicators of AIDS.

All of these patients started with CD4 counts of greater than 300. Dr. Bihari indicates that most patients with lower CD4 counts showed a decline in CD4 number and percentage over time, though much more slowly than untreated patients used to.

> LDN Plus Antiretroviral Therapy

Since the advent of HAART 5 years ago, Dr. Bihari has used it in combination with low dose naltrexone in all of his patients with lower CD4s. As of 2002, nearly all of his 175 patients in this category are on at least one protease inhibitor and either nevirapine or two nucleoside analogues. The group who began 5 years ago numbered 102 patients; there have been 3 dropouts since. There have been at least three interesting findings in this group:

1. **The viral load breakthrough rate in 5 years has been only 14% in the 102 patients who have been taking LDN along with HAART for that full time period. More than 85% have remained HIV RNA-PCR undetectable during this period.** Reports from other treatment groups have shown an average breakthrough rate of 30-50% in the first twelve months, and 60-70% by the end of three years. The only difference in the treatment approach that could explain this is that all of Dr. Bihari's HIV patients are taking low dose naltrexone.

2. **Seventy-five percent of those on HAART and low dose naltrexone, including the few with viral-load breakthroughs, are showing a slow secondary rise in CD4s, which generally begins after 18 months on HAART.** This late rise in CD4s in all cases has been persistent in all cases. In the 99 long-term patients, there has been a mean rise of CD4's from 285 to 496 (87%). This is significantly greater than the rise seen with HAART alone. The medical literature does not appear to have studies showing this phenomenon in patients not on LDN.

3. **None of the more than 175 patients on protease inhibitors have developed any sign of lipodystrophy, except for four who stopped naltrexone.** These are four patients who stopped naltrexone in their early months of HAART, all of whom began to develop lipodystrophy six to nine months later. All four eventually resumed naltrexone. Three experienced complete reversal of lipodystrophy signs after nine or ten months back on the medication. The other has shown significant movement toward reversal at twelve months. Dr. Bihari speculates about the relative role of high cortisol levels and low endorphin levels in the development of lipodystrophy. He suggests that LDN's ability to raise endorphins to counterbalance the cortisol may be responsible for its protective role.

> HIV/AIDS in the Developing World

A new project has been initiated with the cooperation of Dr. Bihari. This aims to acquaint all of the developing nations about the potential of LDN in dealing with the AIDS pandemic.

(Click here for The Developing Nations Project.)

Noteworthy Cases

Examples of patients with successful treatment outcomes, as of December 2001:

(Note: patients listed started naltrexone at the 3mg dosage. Beginning November 2000, all patients switched to naltrexone 4.5mg at Dr. Bihari's suggestion.)

V., a 47-year-old man, was diagnosed HIV-positive October 1989, but did not begin taking LDN until June 1992. In April 1992 he showed a CD4 count of 580 (CD4%=29). In July 1999, after 7 years on LDN with no antiretrovirals, his CD4 count was up, at 776 (CD4%=29.4). His general health status as of an April 2000 office visit to Dr. Bihari was good.

M., a 53-year-old man, was diagnosed HIV-positive in July 1990. He started on LDN January 1991, with a baseline CD4 count of 742. More than 10 years later, his CD4 count was slightly higher, at 778. At his latest office visit to Dr. Bihari, in September 2001, he was found to have mild neuropathy and lymphocytosis. At no time has this patient taken antiretroviral medication.

L., a 37-year-old woman, was diagnosed HIV-positive in March 1992, and began taking LDN 5 months later. Prior to starting on LDN, she took AZT for an unspecified period of time. Her CD4 level, as measured in April 1992, was 321 (CD4%=50.3). Her latest test results, as of June 1999, showed a CD4 level increase to 444 (CD4% had decreased to 42.9). She had never taken antiretrovirals. In her latest office visit to Dr. Bihari (January 2001), she was pregnant and doing well. She recently gave birth to an HIV-negative baby.

S., a 40-year-old man, was diagnosed HIV-positive in 1992, and began taking LDN in December 1993, at which time his baseline CD4 count was 422 (CD4%=20). His latest lab tests, administered December 2001, after 8 years on

LDN with no antiretrovirals, showed a CD4 count of 756 (CD4%=25). His general health status as of his latest visit to Dr. Bihari (December 2001) was excellent.

G., a 48-year-old man, was diagnosed HIV-positive and began taking LDN in May 1997. Measured in March of 1997, his baseline CD4 count was 557 (CD4%=33). His most recent lab test, October 2001, showed a CD4 level increase to 718 (CD4%=42). Health status was good as of a November 2001 office visit. Note: This patient began taking the antiretrovirals Crixivan and Viramune at the same time he started on LDN, but stopped taking them at Dr. Bihari's suggestion after three and a half months.

Example of patient on antiretroviral therapy having prompt response to lipodystrophy when LDN added (June 2002):

M., a 53-year-old woman, not only had diabetes, which required a moderately high dosage of insulin (90 units daily), but also was suffering from lipodystrophy as a complication of her AIDS therapy. In early May, Dr. Bihari noted that he expected LDN would combat her lipodystrophy (which includes insulin resistance) and therefore would probably decrease her insulin needs. Three weeks later, he saw her again for the first time since LDN had been started. Her insulin requirements had dropped from 90 units/day to 20 units/day during those three weeks, and her "buffalo hump" (a swelling at the upper back/lower neck area characteristic of lipodystrophy) had regressed by two-thirds. Her swollen abdomen had begun to recede, enabling her, she said, to cross her legs "for the first time in a year".

What Patients Say

LDN Conference presentation (2006). William Way spoke on the LDN Advocates Panel at the April 2006 LDN Conference on the NIH campus in Bethesda, Maryland. He described having first tested positive for HIV 16 years ago—since that time he has used nothing stronger than nightly LDN to treat the HIV infection. During these many years he reports that his CD4 cell count has, for the most part, remained in a favorable zone, and he has been symptom free. In contrast to virtually any other person who has carried an HIV infection for many years, Mr. Way has never had to use antiretroviral drugs, thus avoiding the attendant expense, annoying schedules, and risk of side-effects.

Phone survey (2001). In November 2001, seven of Dr. Bihari's HIV-positive patients who take LDN without antiretrovirals were interviewed by telephone. Here are some of their responses to the following questions:

How would you describe your experience with using LDN?
How has it been beneficial?
Are there any negative aspects?

"Absolutely positive. There were really no other choices [when I was first diagnosed]. LDN gave me some hope. Over time, my [CD4] counts never dropped. I kept waiting, and they just never dropped. So far, it's been really great. I believe in LDN—it makes sense to me."

"No negative aspects whatsoever. LDN has, I believe, kept my CD4 count from dropping—it has been the same since I started to take LDN (in 1991)… 300 to 350, in that range. I remember when I first started to take it, I felt very different—after a month I felt better all of a sudden. About that time my roommate said to me one day: 'You look so different; you look so much better; your face looks so healthy.' It's been very positive—and it's inexpensive. I believe it's been the major factor in keeping me healthy."

"No negative aspects at all. My viral load has been stable ever since I've been diagnosed and taken this medication. It's been great—no side effects or anything negative about it; everything's been positive."

"I'm basically doing pretty well without being on any of the protease inhibitors ever."

"Sleep was difficult [on LDN] for 2 weeks or a month—I felt buzzy. I learned to take it closer to bedtime, which helped. Only for a short period was this a problem. Benefits: my viral load has regularly been undetectable or negligible. LDN has been very good for me, non-problematic, inexpensive. It seems like it's had a very good effect on my life."

"No negative aspects. My [CD4] numbers have maintained—up around 800 or 900 since day one."

"No negative aspects at all. LDN is what's helped me a lot over the years. I've been HIV positive for almost 15 years now, and have never been sick with any symptoms related to HIV. I think that's mostly because of LDN."

Background

> History

LDN has been in use in the treatment of HIV/AIDS since the completion of a double-blinded placebo-controlled trial in 1986. The trial showed significant immune system protection from HIV in the group given the active drug.

The development of LDN was based on several biological facts. One was the fact that naltrexone, which had been licensed in 1984 as an adjunct in treating heroin addiction, has the ability to induce increases in the endorphin levels in the body. Another was the fact that endorphins are the primary supervisors or (homeostatic) regulators of the immune system, representing 90% of immune system hormonal control. Ninety percent of the day's endorphins are produced by the pituitary and adrenal glands between 2a.m. and 4a.m.

Dr. Bihari and his colleagues then showed that endorphin blood levels averaged less than 25% of normal in people with AIDS. These facts all provided the background for the discovery of the value of LDN in HIV/AIDS. The nocturnal production of endorphins allowed Dr. Bihari and his colleagues to experiment with small doses of naltrexone taken at bedtime in order to jump-start endorphin production. They found that LDN increased endorphin production when taken at bedtime in doses of 1.5mg to 4.5mg. Doses lower than 1.5mg had no effect on endorphin production. Doses higher than 4.5mg produced no more of an endorphin boost, but did block endorphins for significantly longer, thereby reducing the benefit of increased endorphin levels.

Dr. Bihari and his colleagues carried out a placebo-controlled trial of low dose naltrexone in 1985-1986 in 38 patients with AIDS. This followed publication of considerable laboratory research in basic immunology done by Plotnikoff and others that had shown how endorphins play a central role in regulating the immune system. LDN was chosen for its ability to induce increased production in the body of two endorphins, beta endorphin and metenkephalin. A dose was chosen, 3.0 mg at bedtime, that raised endorphin levels without blocking them for more than a few hours. The elevated endorphin levels persisted for 20 to 24 hours.

The 12-week trial showed a significant difference in the incidence of opportunistic infections. There were 5 such infections in 16 patients on placebo and none in 22 patients on the drug. Lymphocyte mitogen responses declined on placebo and not on the drug. Finally, the pathologically elevated levels of acid-labile alpha interferon, present in all 38 patients, declined significantly in the patient group that took LDN and did not drop in those on placebo.[1,2]

After the trial, Dr. Bihari began to use LDN in his private medical practice. He was able to do so because the drug is FDA approved for another use, which is the treatment of heroin addiction at a dose of 50mg/day. In 1995, he evaluated the results associated with the use of naltrexone in 158 patients. Only 10 were on antivirals. The results were quite striking. Patients who had taken the drug regularly as prescribed (compliant) showed no drop in CD4 cells. The average CD4 number in these patients before starting naltrexone was 358, and the average 18 months later was 368. The 55 patients who had not taken the drug, or had taken it only sporadically (non-compliant), showed a drop of CD4's from an average of 297 to 176 in 18 months. This represented a drop of approximately 80 per year, roughly the usual rate of drop in patients with HIV with no treatment. Thus, LDN had completely stopped the CD4 drop. This stabilization of CD4's was accompanied by an arrest of disease progression. The 55 non-compliant patients experienced 25 opportunistic infections, and the 103 compliant patients only 8. Survival was also significantly different between the groups. There were 13 deaths among the 55 non-compliant patients and only one in the group of 103 compliant patients. Some patients in this study had been on naltrexone for as many as 7 to 8 years, with no disease progression or CD4 drop and no evidence of resistance to the beneficial effects of the drug. None of the patients experienced side effects.

Many years later, in 1998, a relevant laboratory research paper was published by Sharp et al in the journal Biochemical Pharmacology. It demonstrated that activation of delta-opioid receptors of acutely infected CD4+ T cells significantly inhibited HIV expression in those cells. [Ed. note: activation of these receptors is one of the effects of the endorphins that are stimulated by taking LDN.] [3] (abstract)

> The 1996-1998 Study

In September 1998, Dr. Bihari reported on his retrospective, private-practice based, observational study of the effects of a combination of highly active antiretroviral therapies (HAART) and LDN on HIV RNA-PCR, CD4 levels, adverse reactions and clinical status in 85 patients with HIV/AIDS.

The study was begun in August 1996 when nevirapine became widely available, 4 to 7 months after the availability of indinavir and two other new protease inhibitors. All 85 of the patients were already on LDN. Based on CD4 levels, clinical history and personal preference, 60 of the 85 were started on or were already receiving lamivudine (Epivir). Forty-nine were also on zidovudine (Retrovir) and 4 on stavudine (Zerit) with lamivudine. Twenty-five received indinavir, nevirapine and naltrexone without other antivirals. Treatment with naltrexone, zidovudine and lamivudine or stavudine always preceded the initiation of indinavir and nevirapine, by 3 to 15 months.

The age range was 22 to 74. Ten were women and 75 were men. Thirteen were African-American, 6 were Latino, and 2 were Asian-American. The mean time from initiation of indinavir and nevirapine therapy to the most recent laboratory results was 20 months. Half of the group had been on this combination for 23 months when the most recent labs were done. Patients who were on O.I. prophylaxes before starting these new antivirals were all continued on them, no matter how great the magnitude of rise in CD4 number and CD4 percentage. All patients were started on 1000 mg of indinavir every 8 hours. This was raised from the usual 800 mg every 8 hours to compensate for nevirapine-induced lowering of indinavir blood levels.

Seventy-five patients became PCR undetectable in 4 weeks and remained so. Six never reached undetectable levels. Three did reach undetectability on only one test but then quickly rose back into the detectable range. These 9 acknowledged significant and prolonged lapses in compliance with the indinavir regimen. Only one compliant patient had a sustained suppression of viral load to undetectable (for 6 months) followed by plasma viremia. Seventy-five had no detectable HIV since the first month's test.[4]

There was not a single major opportunistic infection in the 85 patients. One had an episode of shingles. None had thrush. All but one patient remained at their ideal weights or higher. None died or was lost to follow-up. Most patients noted a significant increase in energy, appetite and mood after adding the antiretrovirals.

Only one case of the lipodystrophy syndrome was observed in this patient group. There were, except for this one patient, no changes in fat distribution, in serum triglycerides, in blood glucose or significant rises in serum cholesterol. Since the range of incidence of this syndrome in other studies of patients on protease inhibitors varies from 11% to 35%, this appeared to be a very unusual finding. The one patient who was an exception supported the likelihood that LDN was responsible for the general protection against the lipodystrophy syndrome.

This patient was on indinavir, nevirapine and LDN for 15 months, with a rise in CD4's, undetectable viral load and no lipodystrophy. He then moved to the west coast of Canada where he was unable to obtain naltrexone, which is not yet a licensed drug in Canada. Because of his sustained viral-load suppression and positive feelings about the new antivirals, he felt the naltrexone was not crucial and discontinued it. About 8 months after stopping low dose naltrexone, he began to develop the changes in body shape associated with lipodystrophy. These physical changes were accompanied by a sharp rise in serum cholesterol, triglycerides and glucose.

Later, Dr. Bihari learned of three other patients who had stopped LDN after starting HAART, then developed lipodystrophy six to nine months later. As mentioned above, three of these four patients experienced clearing of lipodystrophy after nine to twelve months back on LDN.

Footnotes

1. Bihari B, Drury F, Ragone V et al. *Low dose naltrexone in the treatment of AIDS.* IV International Conference on AIDS. Poster 3056. Stockholm, June 1988.
2. Bihari B, Drury F, Ragone V et al. *Low dose naltrexone in the treatment of AIDS: long term follow-up results.* V International Conference on AIDS. Poster M. C.P. 62. Montreal, June 1989.
3. Sharp BM, Gekker G, Li MD et al. *Delta-Opioid Suppression of Human Immunodeficiency Virus-1 Expression in T Cells (Jurkat).* Biochemical Pharmacology, Vol. 56, pp. 289-292, 1998. Read the abstract.
4. Deeks SG, Beatty G, Cohen PT et al. *Viral load and CD4+ T Cell changes in patients failing potent protease inhibitor therapy.* Fifth Conference on Retroviruses and Opportunistic Infections. Abstract 419. Chicago, Feb. 1998.

From LDNINFO.ORG

LDN and Cancer

In Brief

Although prospective, controlled clinical trials on LDN in the treatment of cancer are yet to be accomplished, as of March 2004 clinical "off-label" use of this medication by Dr. Bihari in some 450 patients with cancer — almost all of whom had failed to respond to standard treatments — suggests that more than 60% of patients with cancer may significantly benefit from LDN.

Of the 354 patients with whom Dr. Bihari had regular follow-up, 86 have shown objective signs of significant tumor shrinkage, at least a 75% reduction. 125 patients have stabilized and/or are moving toward remission.

Dr. Bihari's results sharply contrast to prior usual cancer treatment outcomes: either a cancer-induced death or a total cure. LDN therapy presents a viable third alternative, the possible long-term stabilization and/or gradual reduction of tumor mass volume.

Thus, with LDN, cancer can — in some cases — become a manageable chronic disease. Patients have the possibility of living free of symptoms, without, in many cases, the crippling side-effects of chemotherapy and radiation treatment.

> How It Works

Low dose naltrexone might exert its effects on tumor growth through a mix of three possible mechanisms:

1. By inducing increases of metenkephalin (an endorphin produced in large amounts in the adrenal medulla) and beta endorphin in the blood stream;
2. By inducing an increase in the number and density of opiate receptors on the tumor cell membranes, thereby making them more responsive to the growth-inhibiting effects of the already-present levels of endorphins, which induce apoptosis (cell death) in the cancer cells; and

3. By increasing the natural killer (NK) cell numbers and NK cell activity and lymphocyte activated CD8 numbers, which are quite responsive to increased levels of endorphins.[1] (abstract)

> Cancers that are reported by Dr. Bihari to apparently respond to LDN:

- Bladder Cancer
- Breast Cancer
- Carcinoid
- Colon & Rectal Cancer
- Glioblastoma
- Liver Cancer
- Lung Cancer (Non-Small Cell)
- Lymphocytic Leukemia (chronic)
- Lymphoma (Hodgkin's and Non-Hodgkin's)

- Malignant Melanoma
- Multiple Myeloma
- Neuroblastoma
- Ovarian Cancer
- Pancreatic Cancer
- Prostate Cancer (untreated)
- Renal Cell Carcinoma
- Throat Cancer
- Uterine Cancer

> What the Future Holds

If the results of trials of low dose naltrexone in certain cancers are positive, the drug could eventually become an additional mainstay of cancer treatment — adjunctive with chemotherapy, radiation, and other cancer cell growth inhibitor receptor agonists — or even a replacement for current therapies, as primary treatment for those cancers that show little response to standard therapies.

Recent Developments

> As of March 2004

Since February 1999, Dr. Bihari has begun treatment of some 450 cancer patients with LDN. Since many of these patients, particularly those seen before October 2000, were seen only once in consultation with medical follow-up by their oncologists, Dr. Bihari is missing up-to-date follow-up data on 96 patients.

As of March 2004, of the remaining 354 patients, 84 have died, all but 4 of cancer-related causes. Most of these deaths have occurred in the first 8 to 12 weeks on LDN. For the most part, these were patients who were quite ill when first seen, and had exhausted all other treatment possibilities. Of the remaining 270 patients, 220 have been on LDN for six months or longer. Of these, 86 have shown significant movement toward remission, identified for this purpose as a reduction of at least 75% in tumor mass and tumor-related symptoms. Of the other 134 patients, 9 have continued to show tumor progression, whereas the other 125 have stabilized and/or are moving toward remission but do not yet meet the 75% reduction criterion.

LDN and Cancer: Outcomes for 450 Patients as of March 2004

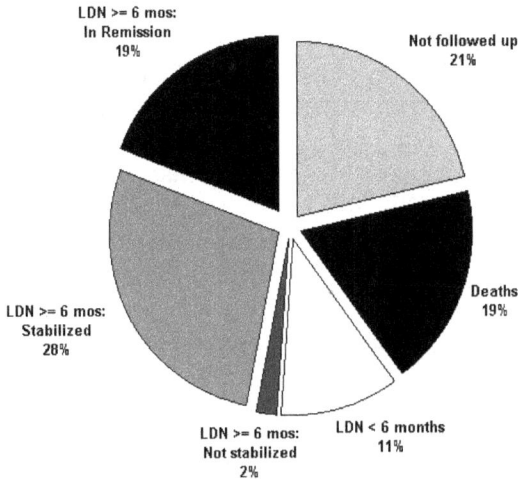

Among those who have shown significant movement toward remission, most had never received chemotherapy. The apparent remissions:

- 2 children with neuroblastoma
- 6 patients with non-Hodgkin's lymphoma
- 3 with Hodgkin's disease
- 5 with pancreatic cancer metastatic to the liver
- 5 with multiple myeloma
- 1 with carcinoid
- 4 with breast cancer metastatic to bone
- 4 with ovarian cancer
- 18 with non-small cell cancer of the lung
- 1 with small cell cancer of the lung
- 5 with prostate cancer (no prior hormone-blocking therapy)

(Although recently-diagnosed prostate cancer patients who have not received other therapies appear to do well on LDN, patients with prostate cancer who have already been treated with hormone-related therapies, including testosterone-blocking drugs and PC-Spes, have not responded to LDN.)

An overview of these results must assume the basic statistical principle that the patients with no follow-up contact have not done as well as those who have maintained continual medical contact with Dr. Bihari. Measured in terms of disease stabilization and/or movement toward remission, and assuming that patients in continual follow-up are twice as likely to have had a good outcome thus far, it appears that over one-half of all cancer patients whom Dr. Bihari has started on LDN have done well.

Taking into account the relatively large number of patients who were in advanced stages of disease when first seen by Dr. Bihari, and that some patients in the "not followed up" and "LDN < 6 mos" groups will likely have positive outcomes, it appears possible that more than 60% of patients with cancer may significantly benefit from LDN. This is underscored by Dr. Bihari's observation that better outcomes tend to be seen when treatment with LDN is begun in earlier stages of the disease. Of interest, there is a negligible rate of relapse in patients who are started on LDN after or during successful initial treatment with surgery (e.g., for breast cancer) or with chemotherapy (e.g., for Hodgkin's disease or non-Hodgkin's lymphoma).

It will clearly require extensive study of LDN in prospective, controlled clinical trials to determine which cancers respond best and which other therapies are complementary to or synergistic with LDN.

> Other Developments

LDN Alone in the Treatment of Cancer. Dr. Bihari now has **88** patients with cancer in complete or partial remission whose improvement appears to be clearly attributable to LDN alone. In contrast, the vast majority of patients who consult with him for cancer tend to be on other concurrent treatments as well, which obviously interferes with drawing conclusions about LDN's role in their improvement. The successful LDN-only group includes five breast cancer patients, one patient who had widespread metastatic renal cell carcinoma, three with Hodgkin's disease and six with non-Hodgkin's lymphoma. Other such cases, some now on LDN for as long as four years, include a score of patients with non-small cell lung cancer, as well as patients with ovarian cancer, uterine cancer, pancreatic cancer (treated early), untreated prostate cancer, colon cancer, malignant melanoma, throat cancer, primary liver cancer, chronic lymphocytic leukemia, multiple myeloma and some others.

NCI Examining LDN Cancer Cases. In June 2002 an oncologist and an oncology physician's assistant from the National Cancer Institute reviewed some 30 charts of cancer patients at Dr. Bihari's office. About half were chosen as appearing to have responded to LDN without question. With patients' permission, copies of these were sent to the NCI for further data collection on its part for consideration for NCI's Best Case Series.

Noteworthy Cases

> As of June 2004

Lung Cancer.

C., a 61 year old woman, previously a heavy smoker, was found to have a lesion in the right upper lobe of the lung in 1999 and a supraclavicular node in April 2001. Biopsy showed that the node was metastatic from the lung tumor. In August 2001 an MRI of the chest showed supraclavicular clusters of nodes and stellate-shaped lesions in the apex of the right upper lobe. She then started taking low dose naltrexone. She began getting quarterly C-T scans of the chest, which have shown no change over the following 40 months. The C-T scan interval was changed to every 6 months. Her most recent C-T scan in the spring of 2004 continues to show no change from the August 2001 films.

Malignant Melanoma.

L. is a 53 year old woman with metastatic malignant melanoma whom Dr. Bihari first saw in August 2000. Her primary skin lesion had been removed from the lower back in late 1976. A lump in the left groin was biopsy positive in December 1977. It appeared to respond to treatment with BCG in a clinical trial in January 1978. She was disease free for 20 years until a cancerous lesion appeared near the site of the original primary. It was removed surgically. She started a melanoma vaccine trial in April 1999 but developed two new skin lesions on the low back over the next six months. In February 2000 a bone scan showed a lesion in the left sixth thoracic rib, with growth evident on a repeat bone scan in April 2000, which also showed further lesions in the left sacrum and the L5 vertebra. She began taking low dose naltrexone in August 2000. She showed no growth of these three bone lesions and no appearance of new lesions over a forty month period since that time. She has remained on naltrexone only.

Esophageal Cancer.

Reverend X is a patient at John's Hopkins Hospital where he received most of his medical care. He first developed problems with digestion and some pain in the mid-chest area with swallowing in April 2002. An upper GI exam in May 2002 showed narrowing and irregularity of the lower esophagus. In June 2002, a C-T scan of the chest, abdomen and pelvis showed a 2cm thickening of the lower esophagus extending into the upper stomach. Also seen were five enlarged nodes in the chest and five in the abdomen. Rev X refused chemotherapy and began low dose naltrexone in August 2002. In the following months his difficulty in swallowing has significantly decreased and his weight has stabilized. He notes an improved sense of well being. He has had no therapy but low dose naltrexone.

Renal Cell Carcinoma. R., a 41-year-old man from Toronto with renal cell carcinoma, with metastatic lesions in his liver and lungs, contacted Dr. Bihari about 36 months ago. His oncologists told him there was no effective therapy available, and he said he was anxious to try treatment with LDN. There was no further contact with the patient until early 2002 when his wife called to thank Dr. Bihari. She said that he was doing quite well and that there had been complete clearing of the metastatic lesions as demonstrated by chest and abdominal CT scans.

Throat Cancer.

D., a 54-year-old man who had cancer of the tonsillar area in his throat along with two large metastatic lesions easily visible in his neck, had refused the extensive head and neck surgery proposed by his physicians. They held out little hope for him. Thirty months ago, Dr. Bihari prescribed LDN. The patient's most recent contact with Dr. Bihari was in May 2004 when he was examined. The primary tumor had decreased by one-third in size and the two neck masses had regressed by about 50%. The patient had received no radiation or chemotherapy but had tried unproven alternative treatments obtained in Mexico.

Non-Hodgkin's Lymphoma.

B., a 75-year-old woman, was diagnosed with non-Hodgkin's lymphoma in January 1999 by a biopsy of an enlarged lymph node in the side of her neck. CT scans showed enlarged nodes in her chest and abdomen, as well as an enlarged spleen. Bone marrow biopsy showed "10% involvement". Her oncologist recommended a wait and watch approach. She started LDN in July 1999. In January 2000, CT of the chest showed an approximately 50% decrease in the size of all the involved nodes. Repeat CT of the chest in November 2000 showed an 80% decrease in total tumor mass.

Prostate Cancer.

M. is a 59-year-old man with prostate cancer, diagnosed with a biopsy and CT scan in September 1999. With no treatment other than low dose naltrexone, after 4 months on LDN his PSA dropped from 6.3 to 3.4. A special ultrasound, performed after 6 months on LDN, showed a 65% shrinkage of the tumor. His PSA remained stable over the following 16 months when he became ill and died of what may have been a cerebrovascular accident.

Pancreatic Cancer.

D. was an 82-year-old woman with pancreatic cancer, treated with surgical removal in April 1999. Scans showed that a tumor mass had reappeared in the pancreatic area in August 1999, and two metastatic lesions were noted in the liver at the same time. She started low dose naltrexone in September 1999 and stopped taking gemcytabine at that time after a short course of four weeks. Some four months thereafter, an MRI demonstrated disappearance of the primary tumor that had previously re-grown, and the liver metastases had cleared entirely. Two months later, D. had a heart attack and died.

Carcinoid.

C. is a 53-year-old woman with carcinoid, a malignancy that generally arises in the appendix or small intestine and spreads to the bones and throughout the abdominal cavity. She started LDN in June 1999. At that time, she had considerable abdominal swelling, diarrhea two to three times a day, frequent episodes of flushing due to the tumor, poor energy and appetite, and significant metastatic spread to numerous bones. No other treatment for the cancer was administered; none was available. By December 1999, much of the cancer-induced swelling of the abdomen had receded, the diarrhea had completely stopped, the flushing had stopped, and the pain in her right elbow, due to a bony metastasis, had markedly decreased. Follow up in February 2001 indicated that she still had some of the above symptoms and, though clinically stable, was not showing further movement towards remission. A telephone follow-up call in April 2004 indicated that she was experiencing only minimal symptoms.

Multiple Myeloma.

W. is a 72-year-old man with multiple myeloma, diagnosed in the summer of 1998 when a medical workup for severe back pain (that occurred while playing golf) revealed fractures of three vertebrae. Tumor was present in several other bones, blood counts were low, and a bone marrow biopsy showed 20%

replacement of normal marrow with myeloma cells. His serum paraproteins were very high, as they often are in people with myeloma, at 12.6 and with no response to high dose chemotherapy. He started LDN in January 1999 and continued intermittent chemotherapy until October 1999. Since then, he had no chemotherapy but remained on LDN daily. There was a gradual normalization of all of his blood counts, as well as a drop in his abnormal serum proteins from 12.6 to a normal level of 1.4. Bone scans showed continued slow healing of affected bones, and two bone marrow biopsies showed no sign of myeloma. He had deferred plans for a high-dose chemotherapy with stem cell transplant procedure which had been earlier, and had decided to "watch and wait" while continuing nightly LDN. He was back to playing golf and tennis regularly, but there has been no contact since early 2003.

Hodgkin's Disease.

H., a 36-year-old RN with Hodgkin's disease, was diagnosed in October 1991 with fevers, multiple infections (including toxoplasmosis of the brain), and a positive lymph node biopsy. She had a brief remission of several months following treatment with antibiotics and chemotherapy. She refused repeat chemotherapy when tumor activity resumed, and she remained ill with fevers and many gradually growing tumor masses (externally and internally) over the next four years. She started LDN in June 1997. No other therapy was provided. By October 1997, her fevers had cleared, all of her external enlarged lymph nodes had shrunk to normal, and all of the enlarged nodes seen in the spring of 1997 on CT scans were gone. She was determined by her oncologist to be in remission. Since that time, she has moved, gotten married, and not returned repeated phone calls. A long term friend reported that she continues to do well except for some persistent memory loss (due to brain lesions associated with her toxoplasmosis). She has stayed on LDN since and, as of the last phone contact in October 2003, had had no sign of relapse.

Non-Hodgkin's lymphoma.

J., a 48-year-old man, had a CT scan in January 1999 because of low back pain after an auto accident. In addition to a bulging disc in his spine, the CT scan showed many enlarged abdominal lymph nodes. Biopsies of nodes in two locations were diagnostic of a non-Hodgkin's lymphoma. The patient refused chemotherapy and treated himself with antioxidants and multiple nutritional supplements. He added low dose naltrexone in October 1999. A repeat CT scan in late January 2000 showed a significant reduction in the size of the pathological nodes, each being reduced in size by about one-third. A more recent CT scan in early August 2003 showed further shrinkage of the enlarged nodes, which were reduced to less than 50% of their original size. The reduction of tumor mass occurred in the absence of chemotherapy or other standard treatments, with low dose naltrexone his only pharmacologic therapeutic agent.

Breast Cancer.

M. is a 41-year-old patient with breast cancer, diagnosed and treated elsewhere in 1998, whose course was complicated by a recurrence involving metastasis to the hip. Outpatient hospice services were sought. Her walking was so badly impaired that she had to be assisted by her friends on her first office visit to Dr. Bihari in June 2000 — at which time she began LDN. She revisited his office in mid-October and reported that she not only was able to return to work but also was well enough to play tennis again. Repeat bone scan in October 2000 showed a 40% reduction in metastatic tumor mass. She then enrolled in an experimental chemotherapy trial at a major cancer treatment center in New York in December of 2001 and died of liver failure on the fourth day of the trial.

Non-small Cell Lung Cancer.

M. is a patient in his late 50's who first visited Dr. Bihari in June 2000. A chronic cigarette smoker, he was told in May 2000 that he had metastatic non-small cell lung cancer. Many abnormal opaque areas had been seen on his chest x-ray, and a biopsy performed on a sizable mass in his right neck had confirmed the diagnosis. He had refused chemotherapy. On examination, he had a 3cm x 4cm x 2cm mass in his right neck. He was started on LDN in mid-June 2000 and, at the beginning of November, revisited Dr.Bihari for the first time. At that time, the patient reported that energy was better and his appetite was good. He had regained 15 pounds, and had returned to working full time. The volume of the neck mass appeared to have decreased by 50%. An MRI exam in November 2000 showed 80% shrinkage of the right neck mass and 20% shrinkage of the masses in both lungs. As of April 2004, the mass in his right neck remained halved in size, with no further growth of his pulmonary lesions.

Ovarian Carcinoma.

V., a 49-year-old woman, first visited Dr. Bihari in early September 2000. She had a five-year history of ovarian carcinoma, with a persistently growing tumor despite repeated courses of chemotherapy and multiple debulking surgery. There was recent increased involvement of the descending colon with the disappearance of formed stools, and she was now experiencing vomiting. Hospitalization was under consideration. She had lost 15 pounds in the two weeks prior to her visit. She was started on LDN at that time, in addition to her existing low-dose Taxol therapy, and within ten days the signs of large bowel obstruction had disappeared. In four weeks, a repeat CA 125 revealed that this tumor marker had dropped from 1600 to 87. Within the first week of November 2000, it was reported down to 42, and her gynecologic oncologist told her that, on abdominal-pelvic examination, he found no masses. She had regained some 25 pounds and felt "wonderful". A repeat MRI showed no visible masses. In March 2001, the CA 125 had risen to 52, then 70, with no return of symptoms or of palpable masses on abdominal and pelvic exams. However, in October 2001 the abdominal masses recurred despite LDN and she died of metastatic cancer four months later.

Background

Before it was first used to treat cancer, LDN had been in use in the treatment of HIV/AIDS. A double-blinded placebo-controlled trial in 1986 showed significant immune system protection from HIV in a group of patients given the active drug. The development of LDN was based on several biological facts. One was the fact that naltrexone, which had been licensed in 1984 as an adjunct in treating heroin addiction, has the ability to induce increases in the endorphin levels in the body. Another was the fact that endorphins are the primary supervisors or (homeostatic) regulators of the immune system, representing 90% of immune system hormonal control. Ninety percent of the day's endorphins are produced by the pituitary and adrenal glands between 2a.m. and 4a.m.

Dr. Bihari and his colleagues then showed that endorphin blood levels averaged less than 25% of normal in people with AIDS. These facts all provided the background for the discovery of the value of LDN in HIV/AIDS. The nocturnal production of endorphins allowed Dr. Bihari and his colleagues to experiment with small doses of naltrexone taken at bedtime in order to jump-start endorphin production. They found that LDN increased endorphin production when taken at bedtime in doses of 1.5mg to 4.5mg. Doses lower than 1.5mg had no effect on endorphin production. Doses higher than 4.5mg produced no more of an endorphin boost, but did block endorphins for significantly longer, thereby reducing the benefit of increased endorphin levels.

During the course of the placebo-controlled trial of LDN in people with AIDS in 1986, a friend of Dr. Bihari's (M.B.) called him when she discovered that she was experiencing an exacerbation of non-Hodgkin's lymphoma which had gone into remission five years earlier after treatment with chemotherapy.

Because of her awareness of the decreased likelihood of a long-term remission with a second round of chemotherapy, she called to ask if his AIDS drug might help her cancer. A recently published study of human lymphoma transplanted into mice suggested that it might. In this study, all of the mice in an untreated group died of lymphoma. A second group of mice was pre-treated with a single injection of beta-endorphin before the lymphoma transplant. Half of this second group did not get ill with lymphoma. The other half of these mice did, but with a much more slowly growing tumor and a much prolonged life span compared with that of the non-pre-treated group.

Dr. Bihari agreed to treat M.B. with LDN, and used the three golf-ball-sized tumors in her groin as markers of response. All three shrank and disappeared over the next six months. M.B. stayed on LDN and had no further exacerbations of her malignancy. She died six years later in her mid-seventies from her third heart attack.

Several months later, Dr. Bihari, while in Paris to present the LDN AIDS results at an International AIDS Conference, met a woman (C.P.) in her early forties who was quite ill with metastatic malignant melanoma. This had spread from a malignant mole on her arm to her brain, which showed four metastases on C-T scan. Her speech was slurred, her balance and handwriting impaired, and she suffered from headache and recent memory impairment. Her oncologist in Paris said the malignancy was untreatable, and believed that she had perhaps three to six months of life remaining. On his return to New York, Dr. Bihari shipped LDN to C.P.'s daughter, who started the patient on it. Nine months later, with all neurological signs and symptoms having cleared, C.P. had a repeat C-T scan that showed no residual tumor.

C.P. remained on LDN for the succeeding 12 years, stopping it without her family's knowledge in late 1999. Until that time, she had remained in complete remission, without any recurrence of her malignancy. Eight or nine months after stopping LDN she developed nodules under her skin and began to cough up blood. A C-T scan of the chest showed multiple metastatic lesions. Biopsy of one of the subcutaneous nodules confirmed recurrence of malignant melanoma. Dr. Bihari shipped LDN to the patient's family and she resumed it in early 2000. Eight months later, the nodules in the skin had cleared and a repeat C-T scan of the chest showed no residual tumor. She appears to be, once again, in remission.

Over the years encompassed by these two cases, 1986 to 1999, Dr. Bihari focused his research energy on the study of LDN's effect on immune function and on immunological approaches to the treatment of HIV/AIDS. In 1999, however, conversations with three small pharmaceutical companies revealed some interest in the development of LDN, with a goal of getting FDA approval for immune-related diseases including cancer. With this development possibility, Dr. Bihari decided to revisit the potential value of treating cancer with LDN.

Dr. Bihari began an informal private-practice-based evaluation of the effects of LDN with a variety of types of cancer in February 1999. He had seen positive results with a small but growing number of patients with cancer during the preceding 14 years, while developing the drug as an immune modulator for HIV/AIDS. The drug was compounded by pharmacists in 3mg capsules and taken once a day at bedtime. Most patients have recently had their LDN dose increased to 4.5mg daily. It is nontoxic and has no side effects. Its only interaction with other drugs is with narcotics (such as morphine, Demerol and Percocet), which it briefly blocks.

> Mechanisms

The mechanisms involved in the apparent beneficial effect of LDN on cancer have three main elements. The first is the effect of LDN, when taken late at night, in inducing a sharp increase in pituitary and adrenal production of beta-endorphin and metenkephalin, respectively, in the pre-dawn hours, when 90% of the day's manufacture of these hormones occurs. Most studies have shown that naltrexone induces a two to three-fold increase in production of metenkephalin, the endorphin that most specifically activates delta-opioid receptors, the primary endorphin-related anti-growth factor on cancer cells. The low dose of naltrexone, which in higher doses would block endorphin and enkephalin action on the receptor, is gone from the body in about three or four hours — whereas the elevated levels of endorphins and enkephalins persist all day.

The second step involved in the anti-cancer effect of these hormones results from *direct* activation of opioid receptors of cancer cells by the increased endorphins. If this activation occurs while the cell is dividing, it dies. In fact, relatively small concentrations of metenkephalin, when added to human pancreatic cancer cells or human colon cancer cells growing in the test tube, have been shown to kill both. The apparent mechanism of cell killing is called apoptosis (programmed cell death). This appears to be one of the mechanisms by which endorphins and enkephalins combat cancer.

A third element, which may play a major role in controlling cancer, involves the cells of the immune system, which is regulated/orchestrated to a great extent by endorphins. In particular, endorphins raise the circulating levels of natural killer cells and lymphocyte-activated CD-8 cells, the two immunological cell types that prevent cancer by killing cancer cells as they arise.

It should be emphasized that Dr. Bihari's patients were all treated in a private practice setting without the scientific rigor of a prospective clinical trial. This precludes any scientific claims about the drug's efficacy in treating any of the above-mentioned types of cancer. The results thus far do, however, raise the possibility that the manipulation of opioid receptors on cancer cells as anti-growth factors through the use of endorphins and endorphin-inducing opioid antagonists may eventually prove to have considerable merit, particularly in view of the many years of published, supportive laboratory research findings.

Those cancer cells that have opioid receptors on their cell membranes, and that may, therefore, respond to LDN, include all of those that arise from the gastrointestinal tract. This includes the mouth, esophagus, liver, pancreas, stomach, small intestine, colon and rectum. Lymph glands and the spleen have large numbers of opioid receptors, suggesting that Hodgkin's disease, non-Hodgkin's lymphoma, multiple myeloma and lymphocytic leukemia should respond to LDN. Other malignancies with sizable numbers of opioid receptors on their cell membranes include breast cancer, neuroblastoma, prostate cancer, malignant melanoma, renal cell carcinoma, glioblastoma, astrocytoma, endometrial cancer and small cell and large cell cancers of the lung.

> Research History

Ian Zagon, Ph.D., whose research group has done much of the basic animal work in the area of cancer treatment and endorphins, showed in 1981 in a mouse neuroblastoma model that very small doses (0.1 mg./kg) of naltrexone, given once a day, inhibit tumor growth, prolong survival in those mice that develop tumors and protect some mice from developing tumors altogether.[2, 3]

Zagon had hypothesized that the small daily doses of naltrexone work to enhance the endorphin-related protective effect against cancer in mice by increasing the number and density of opiate receptors on tumor cells. He hypothesized as well that the increase in endorphins known to be induced by naltrexone might play a part in the protective effect of the small daily dose by working directly on the tumors' opiate receptors.[4]

In 1996 and 1997, Zagon and his co-workers, reported on laboratory research using specially-bred mice that had no immune system (so-called "nude mice"). They transplanted, in separate experiments, human colon cancer and human pancreatic cancer into the animals and compared the growth of the cancer between those mice that received daily injections of metenkephalin and a control group that received placebo. In each experiment, metenkephalin acted as a negative regulator of tumorigenesis and was significantly able to suppress tumor appearance and growth in the treated group.[5]

Of especial importance, in 1996 the same group of researchers demonstrated that by utilizing LDN to induce an intermittent blockade of opioid receptors in similar laboratory animals (nude mice), the growth of inoculated human colon cancer was markedly retarded. "At the time (10 days) when all control mice had tumors, 80% of the mice in the 0.1 mg/kg NTX group had no signs of neoplasia." When measurements of metenkephalin plasma levels were made, the group that received LDN had metenkephalin levels that were elevated 2.5-fold compared with the control group. The researchers concluded that the results suggested "that daily intermittent opioid receptor blockade with NTX [low dose naltrexone] provokes the interaction of opioids and receptors in the interval following drug availability, with opioids serving to inhibit tumorigenicity of human colon cancer".[6]

New findings by Zagon and colleagues at The Pennsylvania State University in Hershey were published in the December 1999 issue of the journal Brain Research. They had identified the specific cell receptor for one of the endorphins, metenkephalin (the levels of which are increased by LDN). Zagon stated that the opioids act as growth inhibitors, as well as neurotransmitters, and that this feature has implications for cancer treatment. Metenkephalin is found in all tissues, and appears to be associated with cells undergoing renewal or proliferation. Zagon's group was described as having mounted Phase I trials using metenkephalin in an attempt to control the growth of pancreatic cancer in humans. Pancreatic tumors appear to have low levels of the metenkephalin receptor. Low peptide [metenkephalin] or [opioid] receptor levels may exist in cancer cells in general since they want to stimulate their own growth, Zagon said.[7]

Footnotes

1. Matthew, PM, Froelich CJ, Sibbitt WL, Jr., Bankhurst AD, *Enhancement of natural cytotoxicity by beta-endorphin*, J Immunol 130, pp.1658-1662, Apr 1983.
2. Zagon IS, McLaughlin PJ, *Naltrexone prolongs the survival time of mice treated with neuroblastoma*, Life Sci 28, pp. 1095-1102, 1981. (Abstract unavailable.)

3. Zagon IS, McLaughlin PJ, *Naltrexone modulates tumor response in mice with neuroblastoma,* Science 221, pp.671-3, Aug 12, 1983.
4. Hytrek SD, McLaughlin PJ, Lang CM, Zagon IS, *Inhibition of human colon cancer by intermittent opioid receptor blockade with naltrexone,* Cancer Lett 101(2), pp. 159-64, Mar 29, 1996.
5. Zagon IS, Hytrek SD, Lang CM, Smith JP, McGarrity TJ, Wu Y, McLaughlin PJ, *Opioid growth factor ([Met5]enkephalin) prevents the incidence and retards the growth of human colon cancer,* Am J Physiol 271(3 Pt 2), pp.R780-R786, Sep 1996.
6. Hytrek SD, et al. 1996.
7. Zagon IS, Verderame MF, Allen SS, McLaughlin PJ, *Cloning, sequencing, expression and function of a cDNA encoding a receptor for the opioid growth factor, [Met(5)]enkephalin,* Brain Res 849(1-2), pp. 147-54, Dec 4, 1999.

Other References

Recant L, Voyles NR, Luciano M, Pert CB, *Naltrexone reduces weight gain, alters "beta-endorphin", and reduces insulin output from pancreatic islets of the genetically obese mice,* Peptides1(4), pp. 309-313, Winter 1980.

Zagon IS, McLaughlin PJ., *Opioid antagonists inhibit the growth of metastatic murine neuroblastoma,* Cancer Letters 21, pp. 89-94, 1983.

Zagon IS, McLaughlin PJ, *Duration of opiate receptor blockade determines tumorigenic response in mice with neuroblastoma: a role for endogenous opioid systems in cancer,* Life Sci 35, pp. 409-416, 1984.

Zagon IS, McLaughlin PJ, *Opioid antagonist modulation of murine neuroblastoma: A profile of cell proliferation and opioid peptides and receptors,* Brain Res 480, pp. 16-28, 1989.

Zagon IS, Hytrek SD, Smith JP, McLaughlin PJ, *Opioid growth factor (OGF) [metenkephalin] inhibits human pancreatic cancer transplanted into nude mice,* Cancer Lett 112(2), pp.167-175, Jan 30, 1997.

LDN and Autoimmune Disease

In Brief

There is growing recognition in the scientific community that autoimmune diseases result from immunodeficiency, which disturbs the ability of the immune system to distinguish "self" from "non-self". The normalization of the immune system induced by LDN makes it an obvious candidate for a treatment plan in such diseases.

The experience of people who have autoimmune diseases and who have begun LDN treatment has been remarkable. Patients with diagnoses such as systemic lupus, rheumatoid arthritis, Behcet's syndrome, Wegener's granulomatosis, bullous pemphigoid, psoriasis, and Crohn's disease have all benefited.

Because LDN clearly halts progression in multiple sclerosis, its use has been more recently extended to other neurodegenerative diseases, such as Parkinson's disease and amyotrophic lateral sclerosis (ALS or Lou Gehrig's disease) whose etiology remains unknown but for which there is suggestive evidence of a possible autoimmune mechanism.

In addition, people with fibromyalgia and chronic fatigue syndrome have had marked improvement using LDN, suggesting that these entities probably have an important autoimmune dynamic as well.

Recent Developments

> Parkinson's Disease

As of September 2003, Dr. Bihari reported that there were seven patients with Parkinson's Disease (PD) in his practice, all of whom have shown no progression since beginning LDN. Indeed, two of them have shown clear evidence of improvement in signs and symptoms.

Two people with PD, the first patients with that disorder known to have been treated with LDN, have had good results that persist after more than two years on LDN. One patient, a man in his mid-60's from New Jersey, had his first annual revisit to Dr. Bihari for a check-up in April 2002. His wife reported that, in contrast to all the other members of his PD monthly group meeting, he seemed to have shown no deterioration in his functional abilities throughout the prior year. On a thorough neurological examination, Dr. Bihari found improvement in some signs of his Parkinson's Disease. Among these was now the absence of the glabellar sign, a primitive reflex that is consistently found in those with PD and which the patient had demonstrated the year before on his initial examination.

Another patient with PD is a 48-year-old male who began LDN in December 2000. Because he was seeing no improvement in his condition (although he wasn't getting any worse), he discontinued LDN in early March 2002. He called Bihari in mid-May 2002 because he was now beginning to see, for the first time in over a year, worsening of his PD symptoms. In those three months, the disease manifested increased tremor and rigidity in the involved arm. He resumed LDN and over the following two months experienced reversal of the progression that had occurred off of the drug. He was also able to reduce his dopamine-analogue medication by two-thirds, relieving the depression that it was producing.

> Amyotrophic Lateral Sclerosis

In the spring of 2002, several people with amyotrophic lateral sclerosis, after reading the material about multiple sclerosis on this website, asked their physicians to prescribe LDN for their ALS. Two patients with advanced disease showed significant improvement in their breathing, as measured by a forced vital capacity (FVC). One had a 25% improvement within two months of beginning LDN and the other 11% improvement. A third patient who also has advanced ALS and an impaired FVC has had significant subjective improvement in his ability to breathe and a reduction in his resting pulse from 96 to the low 80's.

Subsequently, in early fall 2002, the first patient, who had been taking only 3mg of LDN nightly, notified us that both his FVC and that of the second patient, who was using the 4.5mg dose, had reverted to their usual baseline capacities, but that their FVC's appeared to be remaining stable for a prolonged period.

[Ed. Note: Given the repeated demonstration of LDN's efficacy in halting progression in virtually all cases of MS (see LDN and MS), and the possibility of its having a therapeutic effect in Parkinson's Disease and in ALS, it may be timely to consider LDN in treating the full spectrum of neurodegenerative diseases whose etiology is unknown—all of which may well have a significant underpinning of immunodeficiency/autoimmunity causing their neurological syndromes. Alzheimer's disease also suggests itself as an important possibility.]

Noteworthy Cases

> Wegener's Granulomatosis

D. is a 62-year-old male. In February 2000, after 3 years of recurrent upper respiratory symptoms and cough, and more recent difficulty with vision, he was admitted to a Boston medical center because of suspected vasculitis. He had lost energy and could not walk more than ten to fifteen steps without having to rest. The autoimmune disease Wegener's granulomatosis was considered probable, due to an elevated sedimentation rate (80) and a positive Anti-Neutrophil Cytoplasmic Antibody [ANCA] level of 65. In May 2000, nasal tissue removed at surgery confirmed "necrotizing vasculitis ... highly suggestive of Wegener's granulomatosis." He was treated with corticosteroids for nine months, until January 2001. The ANCA test was 1.9 in July 2000, 12 in January 2001 and back up to 40 in May 2001, at which time he was experiencing marked fatigue and upper respiratory symptoms.

D. started using low dose naltrexone (4.5mg) nightly in mid-May 2001. After several weeks he noticed a decrease in congestion and a noticeable increase in overall energy. Subsequent tests of ANCA were 16 in August 2001 and the most recent test of ANCA in late December 2001 was down to 1.0. As of September 2002, he continues to report a high energy level—equal to that prior to disease onset—and he is enjoying his noticeable improvement in overall health.

> Crohn's Disease

As of September 2002, Dr. Bihari was following eight patients with Crohn's Disease on LDN. In all eight cases, within 14-21 days the signs and symptoms of disease activity stopped. All eight had remained stable since anywhere from 2 months to 36 months.

> Rheumatoid Arthritis

Ten patients with this disease have been treated with LDN in recent years. In all ten patients the joint pain and swelling cleared, in some, leaving residual joint distortion. Two of the patients stopped LDN for several weeks because of travel. Both had an immediate exacerbation. One patient who was responding well on LDN had a mild exacerbation during a period of severe marital stress.

> Pemphigoid

K. is an 82-year-old woman who, over a period of three months, developed blisters on her ankles, the soles of her feet, her arms and her neck, which on biopsy proved to be pemphigoid. She was referred to a dermatologist specializing in this disease who treated her with prednisone 40 mg/day, which slowed disease progression but did not clear her blisters. When LDN was added by Dr. Bihari, her blisters cleared and slowly healed over a 6-week period, during which time she slowly tapered her prednisone. On her last visit, she was on both LDN each night and prednisone 5mg every other day with no exacerbation.

Background

Naltrexone was licensed in 1984 by the FDA in a 50 mg dose as a treatment for heroin addiction. It is a pure opiate antagonist (blocking agent) and its purpose was to block the opioid receptors that heroin acts on in the brain. When it was licensed, Dr. Bihari, then involved in running programs for treating addiction, tried it in more than 50 heroin addicts who had stopped heroin use. None of the patients would stay on the drug because of side effects experienced at 50 mg such as insomnia, depression, irritability and loss of feelings of pleasure, all due to the effect of the drug at this dose in blocking endorphins. These are the hormones in the body that heroin resembles. Physicians treating heroin addicts therefore, for the most part, stopped prescribing naltrexone. In 1985, a large number of heroin addicts began to get sick with AIDS—studies showed that 50% of heroin addicts were HIV Positive.

Dr. Bihari and his colleagues decided to shift their research focus to AIDS, in particular focusing on ways of strengthening the immune system. Since endorphins are the hormones centrally involved in supporting and regulating the immune system, levels of endorphins were measured in the blood of AIDS patients. They were found to average only 25% of normal.

Naltrexone, when given to mice and people at high doses, raises endorphin levels in the body's effort to overcome the naltrexone blockade. This drug became the focus of Dr. Bihari's research group. When the group discovered that endorphins are almost all produced in the middle of the night, between 2 AM and 4 AM, the studies focused on small doses (1.5-4.5 mg at bedtime) with the hope that a brief period of endorphin blockade before 2 AM might induce an increase in the body's endorphin production. In fact, the drug did so in this dosage range. It had no effect below 1.5 mg and too much endorphin blockade at doses over 5 mg. A placebo-controlled trial in AIDS patients showed a markedly better outcome in patients on the drug as compared with those on placebo.

During the trial, a close friend of Dr. Bihari's daughter had three acute episodes of multiple sclerosis over a nine-month period with complete spontaneous recovery from each. Because of his knowledge of MS as a neurologist and of recent evidence of an autoimmune component in the disease, Dr. Bihari started his daughter's friend on naltrexone at 3 mg every night at bedtime. She took it for five years with no further attacks. At that point, when a particular month's supply ran out, she stopped it because of some denial that she had MS. Three and a half weeks later, she developed an episode of weakness, numbness, stiffness and spasms in her left arm and resumed LDN, which she has stayed on since. This episode cleared and over the 12 years since, she has had no further disease activity.

The apparent mechanism of action of LDN in this disease parallels that in AIDS and other immune-related diseases. A small dose of the drug taken nightly at bedtime doubles or triples the endorphin levels in the body all of the next day restoring levels to normal. Since endorphin levels are low in people with MS, immune function is poorly orchestrated with significant impairment of the normal immune supervisory function of CD4 cells. In the absence of normal orchestration of immune function, some of the immune system cells "forget" their genetically determined ability to distinguish between the body's 100,000 unique chemical structures (called "self") and the chemical structures of bacteria, fungi, parasites and cancer cells (called "non-self"). With this loss of immunologic memory, some cells begin to attack some of the body's unique chemical structures. In the case of people with MS, the tissue attacked by immune cells (particularly macrophages) is primarily the myelin that insulates nerve fibers. These attacks result in scars in the brain and spinal cord called plaques. LDN in such patients works by restoring endorphin levels to normal, thereby allowing the immune system to resume its normal supervision and orchestration.

There exists a common notion that the immune system in a person with an autoimmune disorder is too strong and, in its exuberance, targets a body tissue for attack. Rather, the evidence is more consistent with autoimmunity resulting from immunodeficiency.[1] Kukreja et al have demonstrated that multiple immunoregulatory T cell defects lie behind Type 1 diabetes both in humans and in non-obese diabetic mice.[2]

Multiple scientific papers from various other research centers have demonstrated that an underlying immunodeficiency is characteristic of any tested autoimmune disease. Examples thus far reported include multiple sclerosis, rheumatoid arthritis, Crohn's disease, and chronic fatigue syndrome.[3, 4, 5]

Sacerdote et al measured low beta-endorphin levels in two animal examples of autoimmune disease — a mouse strain with a lupus-like syndrome and a strain of chicken with an autoimmune thyroiditis.[6] They had significantly lower hypothalamic concentrations of the opioid than normal controls. In each case, the low levels of beta-endorphin were found well before the expression of autoimmune disease. This adds to considerable evidence of a key role for endorphins in regulating immune responses and suggests a therapeutic pathway.

Bihari et al found that a low oral dose of the opioid antagonist naltrexone, when taken at bedtime, led to a doubling or tripling of low levels of circulating beta-endorphin.[7] Bihari has since treated some 100 people with autoimmune disorders. None of them has progressed further while the patient continued taking low dose naltrexone each night at bedtime. Since no side effects are apparently associated with its use, this medication might well be studied as a possible preventive for Type I diabetes in those youngsters with beta-cell autoantibodies.

Footnotes

1. Buckley RH. *Primary Immunodeficiency Diseases Due to Defects in Lymphocytes.* N Engl J Med. 2000; 343:1313-1324.
2. Kukreja A, Cost G, Marker J, et al. *Multiple immuno-regulatory defects in type-1 diabetes.* J Clin Invest. 2002;109(1):131-40.
3. Thewissen M, Linsen L, Somers V, Geusens P, Raus J, Stinissen P. *Premature immunosenescence in rheumatoid arthritis and multiple sclerosis patients.* Ann N Y Acad Sci. Jun 2005;1051: 255-62.
4. Marks DJ, Harbord MW, MacAllister R, Rahman FZ, Young J, Al-Lazikani B, Lees W, Novelli M, Bloom S, Segal AW. *Defective acute inflammation in Crohn's disease: a clinical investigation.* Lancet. Feb 2006;367 (9511): 668-78.

5. Vernon SD, Reeves WC. *The challenge of integrating disparate high-content data: epidemiological, clinical and laboratory data collected during an in-hospital study of chronic fatigue syndrome.* Pharmacogenomics. Apr 2006;7 (3): 345-54.

6. Sacerdote P, Lechner O, Sidman C, et al. *Hypothalamic beta-endorphin concentrations are decreased in animals models of autoimmune disease.* J Neuroimmunol. 1999;97(1-2):129-33.

7. Bihari B, Drury FM, Ragone VP, et al. *Low Dose Naltrexone in the Treatment of Acquired Immune Deficiency Syndrome.* Oral Presentation at the IV International AIDS Conference, Stockholm, Jun 1988.

The 146 page book, *Health Case Studies of Low Dose Naltrexone (LDN) in the treatment of a range of* diseases can be downloaded as a pdf file for free at: http://www.casehealth.com.au/case/pdf/those_who_suffer_much_ldn_book_jul 08.pdf

THOSE WHO SUFFER MUCH KNOW MUCH

© 'Case Health – Health Success Stories', 2006 -*casehealth.com.au Revised – July 2007, July 2008* Cris Kerr, Administrator & Community Health Researcher, 'Case Health-Health Success Stories' website, October 2005, rev July 2007, rev July 2008

The 'Case Health – Health Success Stories' website collects and shares health success stories and case studies attributed to any successful health intervention. Though based in Brisbane, Australia, the site holds stories from all over the world and the service is provided as a community service, free of any charge.

A growing body of compelling testimony

I'm an unqualified community health researcher who first became aware of a drug that can halt or slow progression of Multiple Sclerosis (MS), and enhance prolong quality of life for sufferers, after receiving a story submission in 2003. The drug is naltrexone, and my 'Health Success Stories' database contains a growing body of compelling patient testimony that it works, and it works well - BUT, sufferers can't get it. It's not a cure, and it does not work for everyone, but it does work.

The naltrexone story is a powerful story that must be told and shared

Dr Bernard Bihari's groundbreaking work with naltrexone commenced over twenty years ago and has since resulted in a small but growing number of physicians prescribing **low doses of naltrexone (LDN)** to minimize both progression and symptoms of disease for their patients.

Bihari, who retired from private practice in March 2007, first successfully treated HIV patients, then MS and cancer patients. In the ensuing years LDN has been cited as beneficial across many other diseases such as Autism, Crohn's Disease, Hepatitis B, and a long list of others. If you're wondering how all these diseases are linked, look no further than an errant immune system.

In Scotland, Dr Pat Crowley has been prescribing LDN successfully for some time, and even traveled to New York to interview Dr Bihari for his own documentary. In the USA, Dr Jacquelyn McCandless found LDN benefits Autism and is responsible for the development of the first LDN topical formulation - a cream consisting of emu oil and naltrexone that is applied to the skin to bypass digestive issues. Dr McCandless and her husband are presently in Mali, Africa trialling LDN for HIV.

The number of doctors familiar with, and prescribing LDN is still small but growing. Other early adopter advocates are; Dr Bob Lawrence, Dr Tom Gilhooly, Dr Phil Boyle, Dr Burt Berkson, Dr Terry Grossman, Dr Joseph McWhirter, and Dr Jill Smith; who've championed patient needs and hence have contributed to positive progress for this controversial treatment option.

Due to the wonder that is the Internet, word has spread. A maiden patient conference dedicated to LDN was held in New York in 2005, and has since been followed by now annual conferences held in 2006 and 2007. This year's conference is being held at the USC Health Sciences Campus in Los Angeles, California on 11 October 2008.

Disease sufferers whose progression has been alleviated by treatment with LDN have formed groups dedicated to spreading the word. They strive to help fellow sufferers via information-sharing, emotional support, and fund-raising for clinical trials; the first of which commenced in 2007 at the University of California, San Francisco (UCSF) and was partly funded by a dedicated support group linked to SammyJo's LDNers.org.

Why are Clinical Trials important?

Clinical trials seek to answer the 'who, what, why, where, how, and when' questions that must be addressed to establish patient profile, efficacy, optimum dose and time, and of course, safety. Clinical trials establish evidence of successful, safe outcomes or unsuccessful, unsafe outcomes. Doctors therefore, quite rightly, base treatment decisions on clinical trials because this is at present the safest system to follow, and patients wouldn't want it any other way.

However, due to the absence of clinical trial data, the Low Dose Naltrexone Treatment Protocol has not achieved mainstream scientific acceptance as a treatment option for MS or any of the other diseases it has been benefiting.

Whilst a growing number of doctors are prescribing LDN 'off label', most will not prescribe a treatment unproven clinically.

Naltrexone is only officially approved as a treatment for alcohol or drug dependence at doses much higher (around 50mg), than the very low doses (up to 4.5mg) being prescribed 'off label' for the management of HIV, MS, cancer, Crohn's and other diseases. In many jurisdictions doctors can prescribe this drug 'off label', but only where there is no 'proven' treatment for a particular disease or condition. It's my understanding doctors in most jurisdictions can also prescribe a drug 'off label' as an adjunct that complements a 'proven' treatment - though this increases the risk of medication conflict for the patient.

What's wrong with our 'health system'

Clinical trials are expensive and are typically initiated and sponsored by companies that expect to patent a drug and recoup costs by commercializing the successful results. That's business and that's how it should be. If an organisation is prepared to fund the very high cost of research, development, and clinical trials they're entitled to view the cost as an investment that will turn a profit.

Naltrexone is an old drug. It's well past its patent protection period and is now a 'generic'. A clinical trial of an 'off-patent generic drug' doesn't present an attractive commercial proposition for sponsoring organisations that have traditionally initiated clinical trials -because they can't gain exclusive patent rights, and subsequent profits, from a successful outcome. To this end older drugs are often re-engineered - a molecule changed here and there - new drug, new patent, new price.

Unfortunately, health has morphed into a consumer market. That means, just like every other consumer market, the healthcare industry is 'market driven' in terms of meeting consumer 'supply and demand'. This system assumes health consumers wanting or needing a particular healthcare product that's not presently available, will create sufficient demand to drive commercial enterprises to bring a new product to market that fulfils their unmet need, or in other words, supplies their demand.

Subsequently, the primary driving force for Health Research, Development, and Clinical Trials is the potential for profit - but there's no big profit to be made from trialling a 'generic' drug such as Naltrexone, regardless of the promise it holds to alleviate suffering and deliver economic public health benefits, so nothing happens.

Where does that leave the promise of Naltrexone?

Patient testimonies crediting LDN for improved health have been growing exponentially, and a large body of stories from MS sufferers who've slowed or halted progression of their disease or had symptom improvement with LDN are building a compelling case - but these testimonies represent only one facet of evidence. At present, health success stories alone aren't sufficient evidence for most doctors to prescribe LDN.

A large body of health success stories, however; can provide sufficient evidence to advocate for governments to initiate and fund clinical trials, and; when health success stories are recorded in greater detail and numbers as case studies, they can also build into statistically significant volumes of evidence through the sheer power of numbers, achieving 'volume value' in their own right, and facilitating insights into public health priorities and improvement opportunities.

So how did we discover Naltrexone holds such promise?

In New York, USA in the 1980s, Dr Bernard Bihari was focused on improving outcomes for his patients. His research led him to Dr Ian S Zagon's promising lab research with naltrexone in mice with cancer. Bihari began trialling lower doses of naltrexone, resulting in the successful treatment of HIV, then later MS and Cancer.

In the USA, Dr David Gluck, a childhood friend of Dr Bihari and LDN advocate, manages the website lowdosenaltrexone.org and it's sub-site ldninfo.org with the help of his son, Joel. The website features the Foundation for Immunologic Research (FFIR), founded in 1989 by Bernard Bihari, MD and two colleagues in an attempt to raise trial funds for the broader range of LDN's promising applications.

In the UK, LDN Research Trust was founded in May 2004 by Linda Elsegood. Linda is an MS sufferer who's benefited from LDN, and her monthly newsletter features other LDN testimonials. The patients who've been helped by LDN are doing what they can to raise awareness and funds for clinical trials … the hard way.

You can't help but be impressed when you see sufferers of a range of diseases raising funds and contributing to support groups, in spite of their own daily health challenges, in the interest of helping other sufferers benefit from LDN.

Please pause to fully digest what all this means:

Even though benefits were first discovered over twenty years ago, well before any drug was developed to specifically treat HIV or MS, LDN is still not readily available as a treatment option. To my knowledge, this is one of the most powerful examples of the downside of a fully commercialized health market, and why 'balance' must be restored and monitored.

Those that could be helped are not being helped

Whilst there's growing testimony LDN could be the most effective and economic treatment option in the management of MS, HIV, and other diseases (for both the patient and the health system), the absence of clinical trial data means the majority of practitioners are still not prescribing LDN.

Years have passed. Those that could have been helped have not been helped, and those who've exhausted all other treatment options will still not hear of LDN.

What's Disturbing about this Picture of Health?

When you read LDN stories on my website or others I've referenced; the first thing you'll notice is a consistent thread of optimism running through this ever-growing body of health successes:

' ... *I have been on LDN for a little over 7 months now and it has given me a lot of my life back. For the first time in many years, the progression of disability has stopped.* ... '

' ... *I have had NO new symptoms and NO further progression since starting LDN six years ago. I still drive and do all my own shopping, cleaning, etc. I feel certain, had I not been on LDN, I would not be as active as I am, nor as mobile. I wish every MSer had the chance to try LDN to see if they are one of the ones who would benefit.* ... '

The second thing you'll notice is the extraordinary difficulty MS sufferers experience when seeking to trial this treatment. MS is a debilitating condition with multiple adverse symptoms. People with MS are already suffering. You can't help becoming indignant at this injustice:

' ... *I phoned the neuro ... to see if she would give me the Low Dose Naltrexone (LDN) treatment. She had never heard about it ... she was so excited about this ... she had to clear it with the legal dept ... A week later she phoned to tell me the lawyers said no! ... My health was being decided by a group of lawyers!! ... September 4, 2005: I am happy to report a small but significant improvement. Last night for the first time in years I was able to lift my left foot and take a couple of heal to toe steps... instead of dragging my foot or walking toe to heal. ...* '

Patients Abandoned

Dr Bernard Bihari's patients had professional support when they first commenced LDN treatment. This meant, even though his patients had never heard of LDN, they were told what to expect, and were prepared, monitored, and supported by a professional. If an MS patient experienced an exacerbation (with accompanying apprehension) in the first three to six months of treatment, they were likely comforted by; 'this can happen, but experience has shown it does pass'.

Few doctors have knowledge of LDN, and many patients have been abandoned after their doctors learned they were taking LDN - a patient abandoned by her Oncologist, and MS patients abandoned by their Neurologists. Patients returning to their doctors after improvement have been told their initial diagnoses may have been incorrect or their MRIs may have been misinterpreted.

Even more astonishingly, patients who've experienced improvement have been advised to 'keep doing whatever it is they're doing', without any enquiry as to what that may be – not what you'd expect from an enquiring scientific mind focussed on achieving successful health outcomes for their patients.

© 'Case Health – Health Success Stories', 2006 -*casehealth.com.au Revised – July 2007, July 2008*

Page 8/146

Patients without professional support have had to back-fill the knowledge gap and support themselves. This absence of support has resulted in some patients taking LDN without any prior research, knowledge or preparation, and subsequently, with unrealistic expectations.

High expectations, little or no knowledge of what to expect, and no professional support has led to unnecessary angst and disappointment. Subsequently, some who may have benefited from LDN have not, whilst others fortunately, found patient champions within the Yahoo lowdosenaltrexone patient discussion group and were eventually guided to success.

Dr David Gluck's ldninfo.org website contains a wealth of information to aid research and preparation, yet there are still those who begin LDN in haste, who commence LDN concurrently with other medications that conflict, or who defer complementary lifestyle changes such as modifying their diet or alcohol intake, or supplementing nutritional or dietary deficiencies.

I've been observing communication exchanges within the Yahoo LDN group for years now, and it's provided many insights: Those who patiently research and prepare prior to starting LDN are those most likely to succeed. In fact, patients taking ownership of their own health future has not all been bad news: Researching LDN has often resulted in patients initiating lifestyle improvements that complement and enhance their likelihood of success – and this positive turning point to overall improved health has resulted in additional symptom improvement.

LDN is not a high impact treatment. It can take six to twelve months to benefit progressive forms of MS. Testimony of long-term outcomes varies - from halted disease progression with some reversal of symptoms, to slowed progression with minor symptom improvement such as improved bladder control.

This is where case studies reveal their value, because they provide insights into factors other than LDN that may be contributing to improved outcomes or alternatively, contributing to unsuccessful outcomes - all of which have potential to enhance the likelihood of success for others who follow.

Where's the official body that acts on behalf of patients?

Research, drug development, and clinical trials are initiated by commercial sponsors. That's okay, but there's no recognized impartial body that can officially step up to the plate to speak and act on behalf of (advocate for) all patients. I know this because I've tried, without success, to find an authority that's sanctioned to do so.

Officially recognized specialist 'societies' and 'associations' that should be acting on behalf of patients are often sponsored by organisations that are, as mentioned earlier, commercially and/or politically motivated and therefore, have little incentive to recognize, investigate, advocate, or champion the extended benefits of a generic, unprofitable drug on behalf of patients.

Doctors do record successful health outcomes in detail, but it takes time. At present, the primary motivation to devote that time is the chance of; a) publication in a prestigious scientific journal, or; b) an invitation to present at a commercially-sponsored scientific conference.

In both instances there's little incentive for doctors to devote time to recording successful outcomes from 'generic' drugs that won't enhance sales of patented, profitable drugs, or open pathways to new commercial markets within the multi-billion dollar health industry.

The present system is unjust

The present system is clearly imbalanced and unjust. It's inequitable. It doesn't place sufficient value on health success. It doesn't place sufficient value on advocating for the patient. It doesn't place sufficient value on the need for patient-driven research or clinical trials. If it did, there would be a body sanctioned to speak and act on a promising body of testimonials.

How many stories similar to the LDN story are out there? We don't know, because they haven't all been collected, stored, and shared centrally. That makes me feel uneasy and should make you feel uneasy.

Patient testimony can become evidence through 'volume value'

Recording patient testimony in a structured and meaningful way is important.

Testimonies scattered across the Internet may build awareness, but they can be easily devalued and dismissed as random patient anecdotes. They don't register on the public health radar, can't be validated or measured, are not considered evidence, and don't help build a compelling case.

A collection of health success stories presented as 'case studies' can build into a compelling body of evidence that can no longer be ignored. The collective is greater than the single, and though the LDN story is already an excellent example of the power of numbers, it is still in need of greater patient support.

It's my hope the scientific community will one day be compelled by this volume of corroborating case studies to recognize patient testimony can achieve 'volume value' in its own right.

Governments need to acknowledge the value of patient testimony

The collective LDN story is an excellent example of why 'health systems' worldwide need to balance the scales in favour of patients and give more weight and credibility to patient testimony.

It's my hope governments worldwide, presently reviewing and implementing longer-term visions for improving population health, will welcome, accommodate, and integrate patient testimony as a valued, protected, and integral part of their public health IT systems, and will create official bodies and processes chartered to act on behalf of patients and their evidence - impartially, and without prejudice or conflict of interest.

I am but an individual without sufficient resources to lobby for action on this international human rights issue, this orphan desperately in need of more champions - hence this free book in the hope of building international awareness and support.

He who suffers much will know much - Greek proverb

The US System to Develop Important Health Treatments at Low Cost is Being Hoodwinked

By Dr. David Gluck, M.D.

As a Board-certified specialist in both Internal Medicine and in Preventive Medicine, the continuing availablility of newly effective medical therapies – treatments to help deal with the problems of devastating disorders such as cancers, HIV, or autoimmune diseases – is a critical issue, not only for those patients who are immediately effected but also for their families and for society in general.

Recent years have demonstrated that the methods we had taken for granted, the unswerving commitment of the pharmaceutical companies to develop more effective treatments, is no longer the case.

Within the past month, I contacted the Medical Director of a pharmaceutical company that had recently had an article about its own new drug use published within the New England Journal of Medicine. I told him of the continued excellent results with an unusual medication that he had been first told about in the 1980's. Recently, because of contributions by individuals, this off-label medication had been able to accomplish a small but positive study at Penn State in 2007 on Crohn's disease, and in 2008 two new important studies will be published, one from Milan, Italy and one from the University of California in San Francisco, both on its usefulness in treating multiple sclerosis.

The drug, low dose naltrexone [LDN], is available as an off-label prescription. It is generally taken orally as a 4.5mg capsule once a night at bedtime. Naltrexone itself at 50mg was FDA approved in the early 1980's as a treatment for heroin abuse. It is off patent and is a generic medication. The Medical Director told me that he has no problem with the question of efficacy of LDN, he knows it works quite well, his problem lay in convincing his Board that they should lay out 10 or 20 million dollars for a clinical trial for FDA approval and thus risk that the company makes no profits from that cost because anyone can obtain the original drug as a liquid and be able to have the small dose that way.

Therefore, under our present system, millions of people who would have benefited from this inexpensive medication, which has absolutely no toxicity and virtually no side effects, will never discover this brilliant medication, which acts by strengthening one's immune system. LDN thus far has demonstrated its ability to halt the further progression of *any* autoimmune disease (such as rheumatoid arthritis, Crohn's disease, systemic lupus erythematosus, multiple sclerosis, etc.), and often has considerably useful effects on any cancer or HIV infection. In addition, many people with Parkinson's disease and motor neuron diseases (including ALS) have reported improvements or a halt in progression through taking LDN, and a specialist in Neurology has discovered that some 75% of families whose children with autism use it are reporting impressive changes in the child's willingness to play with others.

- There is no question in terms of LDN's efficacy. Unquestionably positive reports, both small studies and scientific trials, are continuing to find their way into esteemed peer-reviewed medical journals – and that information joins with over 20 years of strongly supportive anecdotal reports. See "Clinical & Animal Trials of LDN" at www.ldninfo.org.

- From the first, FDA approval of LDN's special uses has been blocked, perhaps unintentionally, by the existing system in the which sets up the large well-financed pharmaceutical firms as the virtual "gatekeepers". Given that the existing system is based on the legal approval of each newly proposed drug by the FDA, and that the FDA requires clinical trials' results of great cost, it is only the funding pharmaceutical companies' determination of *the potential profitability of any individual candidate drug, no matter its potential therapeutic usefulness*, which decides whether a new medication will or will not have an opportunity to reach the public marketplace and thus contribute to the public health.

- Thus, the stated health-related mission of a pharmaceutical company is generally not at all compatible with that of its necessary primary motivation, which is to gain earnings and profits. This leads to an erosion of medical advances, paradoxically in an era of severely mounting medical costs, in that *an off-patent generic drug with a newly found usefulness, which could significantly heal the sick and/or prevent further illness, even while substantially reducing health care costs, is for all intents and purposes, made unavailable by our system to the public because of its low profit potential.*

- In order to remedy this system of non-performance, and to permit governmental agencies to truly serve the health of the citizenry, *systematic change is called for*. Some key elements of suggested change:

> An Institute of Medicine [IOM] shall be empowered to become the health "czar", overseeing certain major decisions concerning all new medical treatments and devices. It may overrule the FDA when it deems necessary. The new IOM will be sufficiently funded and staffed to be able to arrange support for any and all necessary clinical trials it deems of value, and it shall choose those appropriate centers of excellence at which such studies shall be performed.

> The managing committee of the IOM shall be retained and remunerated in a fashion parallel to that of the Supreme Court, and members shall hold their assignments (unless duly impeached) until a preset age (? 75yo) or until resignation. No member shall be permitted to join with or consult for any commercial pharmaceutical company in any capacity at any time during, or forever after, his or her IOM tenure.

> Members shall be nominated by the President of the , and each must be duly confirmed, if feasible, by the Senate, as entirely disinterested medical academics and research experts of the finest reputations. Highest qualifications must be sought in all cases, and a member's commitment to the highest goals for the public's improved health at the most reasonable cost is mandatory.

> A mandated function of the IOM must include the continual screening of all submitted ideas for improved treatments from medical practitioners and from the general public. Summary reports and comments shall be published at least at monthly intervals throughout the calendar year. Significant penalties for staff performance inadequacy in this area will be mandatory. Exclusive attention to ideas generated by known medical research centers shall be carefully avoided.

> It is expected that, other than as above provided, current functions of the NIH, CDC, Attorney General and FDA should be generally unimpaired by this new system, with which they will cooperate, and which will be devoted to serving the development of new, useful, and cost-saving therapies for the public health in a truly disinterested manner.

> Let us hope that there are enough representatives in government who will see the importance of our country having other than its current "free market system", which is devoted

to pharmaceutical profits, but rather a medical commitment to the discovery of new and unfettered treatments at the lowest prices.

From GAZORPA.COM

The History of Naltrexone

Naltrexone, short for Naltrexone Hydrochloride (C20H23NO4-HCl), is an opiate antagonist. At a therapeutic dose of 50mg per day, Naltrexone blocks the parts of the brain that "feel" pleasure when a person uses alcohol or narcotics. When these areas of the brain are blocked, a person feels less need for "one more drink" or "one more hit."

FDA-approved for the treatment of alcohol and opiate abuse, Naltrexone has recently shown great promise in the treatment of other medical conditions.

The Beginnings

Naltrexone was originally synthesized in 1963 and patented in 1967 as "Endo 1639A" (US patent no. 3332950) by Endo Laboratories, a small pharmaceutical company in Long Island, NY, a company with extensive experience in narcotics.

In 1969, DuPont purchased Endo Labs. DuPont had been struggling to develop its drug business since the late 1950s, and the acquisition of Endo provided DuPont with valuable expertise in drug manufacturing and marketing.

In the purchase, DuPont acquired the rights to several successful Endo drugs, including: Coumadin (warfarin), an anticoagulant; Percodan, a prescription narcotic; and Naloxone, a drug used for narcotic overdose.

Naltrexone, still in its early development phase, came to DuPont as part of the overall purchase of Endo.

At the time it seemed unlikely that DuPont would develop naltrexone, because at the time, naltrexone seemed to have relatively low market potential, and its patent would probably expire before the completion of any clinical trials.

The Federal Government Steps In

In June 1971, President Nixon created the Special Action Office for Drug Abuse Prevention (SAODAP). The first director of SAODAP, Dr. Jerome Taffe, was determined to improve access to drug abuse treatment by shifting services from prisons and hospitals to community-based services. "I regarded the development of naltrexone as one of my high priorities," said Dr. Taffe.

SAODAP recognized that the development of naltrexone was of no burning interest to the private pharmaceutical industry, and that governmental funding would be necessary to bring it to market.

In March 1972, Congress passed the Drug Abuse Office and Treatment Act, calling for development of "long-lasting, non-addictive, blocking and antagonist drugs or other pharmacological substances for the treatment of heroin addiction." This Act provided substantial financial support for research.

By mid-1974, as SAODAP began to phase out of existence, the narcotic antagonist development project fell to the newly formed National Institute on Drug Abuse (NIDA). That same year, NIDA approached DuPont with the idea of developing naltrexone as a drug addiction therapy, and asked for DuPont's assistance in facilitating naltrexone's transit through the FDA approval process. DuPont agreed to assist NIDA with the development of naltrexone. In return, NIDA agreed to pay for the bulk of clinical development costs.

When asked later, DuPont representatives said that the primary reason for helping the government was Dupont's "public spirit", and that naltrexone would probably not have been developed without the government's clinical and financial support.

The clinical trials for naltrexone as a treatment for heroin addiction began in 1973 (Schecter 1974, O'Brien 1978).

Difficulties in Clinical Trials

Early trials of naltrexone in rats, rabbits, dogs and monkeys had determined that the drug was nontoxic at therapeutic levels, with very few side effects. The subsequent human trials confirmed that the drug was safe for humans, but the efficacy trials ran into some unexpected problems.

Dr. Arnold Schecter, who conducted many of the early studies, reported that many opiate-addicted patients feared a new drug, lacked a desire to become drug free, were unwilling to possibly receive a placebo, and disliked the rigid protocols associated with the clinical trials (Schecter 1980).

Patients had to remain opiate-free for a minimum of 5 to 10 days prior to treatment because naltrexone causes severe withdrawal symptoms in patients with opioids in their system (Schecter 1974). Many addicts were unable to comply, due to the physiological effects of withdrawal.

Taking naltrexone does not provide any drug reinforcement ("high"), and produces no negative consequences (withdrawal) when discontinued. Unlike methadone, which helps suppress cravings, naltrexone has no effect until the addict attempts to use heroin. Some patients feared naltrexone would make them more vulnerable to these cravings, and felt that methadone was more effective in controlling them.

Because of these recruiting difficulties, researchers made no effort to screen out patients who might be difficult to manage in clinical trials -- e.g., patients who were poorly compliant -- and this may have compromised the results of the trials (Schecter 1980).

Since naltrexone is non-addictive and lacks the reinforcing effect of methadone, it requires more extensive psychosocial support services than methadone. Support services are expensive. Schecter estimated that total clinical treatment with naltrexone was almost twice as expensive as methadone -- not because of the medication itself, but because of the more intensive support services.

Early trial results showed that, compared with the methadone patients, the patients who were attracted to naltrexone therapy were relatively "more motivated and emotionally stable." Other studies showed that

although naltrexone was an effective opiate block, clinical success (a reduction in heroin use), was limited to fully compliant patients.
As a result of these findings, the product labeling for naltrexone reads, "[Naltrexone]…does not reinforce medication compliance and is expected to have a therapeutic effect only when given under external conditions that support continued use of the medication".

The final results of the clinical trials showed that naltrexone was modestly successfulin the reduction of heroin use.

In 1984, the FDA approved naltrexone in a 50mg dose as a treatment for heroin addiction. Dupont brand-named the drug Trexan.

The same year, DuPont's naltrexone patent expired.

On March 11, 1985, the FDA designated naltrexone as an orphan drug,** which provided seven additional years of market exclusivity for naltrexone for DuPont.

Marketing Strategy for Trexan

The DuPont sales force had trouble explaining the mechanism of naltrexone and its benefits to a lay audience. The consumer marketplace had many misunderstandings and negative perceptions about naltrexone. One former member of the DuPont sales force said these misunderstandings were a great barrier to the use of Trexan.

DuPont also had an extremely difficult time trying to convince methadone clinic personnel to use Trexan. Most facilities could not afford to implement Naltrexone therapy due to the combined price of the drug, the drug treatment program, and the additional time and staff necessary for psychosocial counseling.

Methadone clinics were also reluctant to refer patients for Trexan because of their need to keep their own censuses high enough to receive funding (Schecter 1980).

Pro-methadone treatment providers argued that because methadone was dependence- producing, it was easier to maintain a patient on Methadone, and thus more likely that treatment would be successful.

As a result of these problems, Trexan failed to penetrate the highly regulated federal treatment market for opioid addiction.

By 1995, Trexan sales were approximately $5-8 million annually, which represented approximately 15-25,000 patients per year, or less than 5% of the estimated number of heroin addicts (Scrip 1993).

Naltexone as a Treatment for Alcoholism

Dr. Joseph Volpicelli first recognized naltrexone's potential to treat alcoholism while experimenting with rats as a graduate student in University of Pennsylvania.   In 1981, he began to publish his findings.

In 1985, Volpicelli and Dr. Charles O'Brien, a professor at Penn and chief of psychiatry at Philadelphia's Veterans Administration Center, began a naltrexone study using volunteers at the Veterans Administration Hospital.

"We did it without any outside funding," says O'Brien. "We got it started against pretty great odds." According to O'Brien, the researchers had difficulty recruiting subjects because the idea of treating alcoholism with medication was not commonly accepted in the 1980's.

They tracked 70 men for 12 weeks in an outpatient detox program. Half received naltrexone, half a placebo. While 54% of the volunteers who received a placebo reverted to drinking, only 23% of those who took naltrexone experienced a relapse.

In 1991, researchers at Yale University School of Medicine tested the effects of naltrexone in conjunction with psychological therapy in 104 alcohol-dependent men and women. Patients who took naltrexone were nearly twice as successful in their clinical outcomes as those who took a placebo.

After the Penn and Yale studies were published in the Archives of General Psychiatry in November 1992, DuPont showed interest in marketing naltrexone specifically as an alcoholism treatment.

Governmental funding for the development of naltrexone as a therapy for alcoholism was provided by the National Institute on Alcohol Abuse and Alcoholism. The FDA modified existing regulatory requirements to encourage DuPont to develop naltrexone as an alcoholism therapy.

They offered DuPont three additional years of post-approval market exclusivity for naltrexone as an alcohol therapy.

Marketing exclusivity allows a pharmaceutical company to sell its drug for a certain length of time free of competition from generic versions of the drug. This type of marketing exclusivity is often granted to encourage pharmaceutical companies to develop a use for a drug whose patent has expired or to encourage a company to develop an already approved drug for a new use. With market exclusivity, the expected returns are higher, thus improving the profitability of the drug.

The FDA also linked phase IV clinical trial requirements to annual sales. No phase IV trials would be required if naltrexone as an alcoholism therapy did not meet certain sales thresholds. If the drug did well in the alcohol-abuse market, DuPont would have to conduct phase IV trials based on the level of sales.

By allowing for flexible phase IV studies, the federal government lowered post- marketing costs, improved profitability projections, and made investment in Naltrexone as an alcoholism therapy more attractive to DuPont.

Clinical Trials

Clinical trials for naltrexone as an alcoholism therapy encountered familiar problems -- difficulties with patient recruitment and compliance, high cost of clinical support services, and low funding of treatment centers.

Because researchers had difficulty recruiting patients, they accepted all patients who agreed to participate, and didn't reject any unsuitable patients. This may have negatively affected the results of the clinical trials by including a high proportion of high-risk patients, who may have been motivated more by payment for participating in the trial than a desire for treatment, which led to poorer compliance and higher drop-out rates (Schecter 1980).

The study found that naltrexone as an alcoholism therapy did not perform significantly better than a placebo unless it was administered as part of a comprehensive, multidisciplinary treatment program (O'Malley 1995).

Although the government funded and supported the clinical trials, the funding fell short of the amount necessary to provide the necessary intensive psychosocial support. As a result, the labeling for ReVia (the brand-name eventually chosen by DuPont) includes the following stipulation, "ReVia should be considered as only one of many factors determining the success of treatment of alcoholism." Understandably, this labeling had a profoundly negative effect on marketing strategy and sales.

In 1995, the FDA approved naltrexone in a 50mg dose as a treatment for alcohol abuse. The FDA surprised the researchers by authorizing naltrexone's use in alcoholism treatment in just six months. According to Volpicelli, the FDA was "pretty confident" that the drug was safe: It had been researched for 20 years and was on the market for 10 as a treatment for heroin addiction.

At this point, Dupont changed the brand name from Trexan to ReVia (pronounced "REV-ya"..

Marketing Strategy for ReVia

Because the alcohol treatment system is less regulated than the heroin treatment system, DuPont had more flexibility in marketing ReVia directly to clinics and treatment providers. Despite ReVia's clinical effectiveness and less restrictive distribution channels, however, DuPont's sales force encountered marketing problems.

Like Trexan, ReVia is most successful in highly motivated patients who have a strong psychosocial support and access to counseling services.

DuPont was not successful in selling ReVia, except in comprehensive alcohol treatment programs such as VA hospitals and "white collar" treatment centers. These patients tended to be more highly motivated and have a stronger support network. ReVia became the treatment of choice for more upscale patients, such as physicians, nurses, pharmacists and attorneys (O'Brien).

Another roadblock to naltrexone's wider acceptance was insurance regulations. "Insurance companies often don't allow naltrexone to be prescribed by a primary care physician," said Tania Graves, spokeswoman for the Arizona Medical Association.
"Their point of view is that drug or addiction problems should be sent to a specialist."

Some insurance companies do not accept naltrexone at all. For example, a chain of California treatment centers using naltrexone as the primary treatment had to suspend operations after only six months, citing managed care companies' unwillingness to cover the treatment (Behavioral Health Treatment 1996).

Some physicians were reluctant to prescribe naltrexone due to the "black box" warning of liver toxicity in the package insert. The warning was included based on liver enzyme elevations reported with the100-300mg/day dose (the recommended dose is 50mg) that was given during a study of naltrexone treatment for obesity. A review of literature and adverse effect reports from Dupont demonstrates that a 50 mg/day dose poses no risk for liver damage, but the warning remains (Galloway).

From the American Council on Alcoholism website, 2005:

> Many physicians and non-physicians in treatment programs are unaware of the usefulness of naltrexone or how to use it. In other areas of medicine, it is highly probable that the development of such an efficacious medication would prompt physicians to use it readily. The biggest obstacle to using naltrexone for the treatment of alcoholism is the 'pharmacophobia' of many alcoholism-treatment professionals. This near-hysterical resistance to medication for treating alcoholism (or other substance-abuse disorders) has deep and tangled roots. Many recovering professionals learned in their recoveries that MDs and their prescription pads were evil purveyors of pharmacological lies and temptations. This attitude is often accompanied by a deeply rooted and strongly held belief that recovery has only one successful formula (usually the 12-step program) and that any modification to that approach is unethical.

Scientific evidence is irrelevant to these individuals. They believe they have the 'truth' about recovery and don't want to be bothered with other points of view. [http://www.aca-usa.org/pharm2.htm]

Poor Sales

DuPont never expected either Trexan or ReVia to become major revenue generators, but sales fell far short of even DuPont's modest expectations. In 1994, just prior to the launch of ReVia, Trexan sales were approximately $5-8 million annually, which represented approximately 15-25,000 patients per year, or less than 5% of the estimated number of heroin addicts in the US (Scrip 1993).

When ReVia was launched in January 1995, DuPont expected US sales of ReVia to rise to $15-25 million annually. As of October 1996, however, ReVia had not even reached the FDA's threshold of the 200,000 prescriptions required to trigger phase IV clinical trials (Pink Sheet 1996).

In 1997, ReVia's market exclusivity agreement lapsed. Other companies were now free to manufacture and market generic naltrexone.

In May 1998, the first generic version of ReVia was produced by Barr Laboratories in Pomona NY. At this time, ReVia had annual sales of approximately $20 million.

In 2001, Bristol Myers Squibb acquired DuPont Pharmaceuticals. In April 2002, Bristol Myers Squibb sold the ReVia brand-name rights in the U.S. and Canada to Barr Laboratories.

As of February 2005, Barr manufactures ReVia in 50mg pills in the U.S and Canada. Bristol Myers Squibb continues to market ReVia in countries outside of the U.S. and Canada.

Other versions of naltrexone are currently manufactured in the U.S. by Eon Labs and Amide Pharmaceutical; Mallinckrodt Pharmaceuticals manufactures 50mg and 100mg naltrexone pills in the U.S. under the trade name Depade.

Other 50mg versions of naltrexone are named Nalorex (manufactured by Bristol-Myers Squibb in the UK); Nodict (manufactured by Sun Pharma in India); Naltima (manufactured by INTAS in India), Narpan (by Duopharma in Malaysia), Antaxone (by Pharmazam in Spain), Celupan (by Lacer in Spain), Narcoral (by Siton in Italy), Nemexin (Bristol Myers Squibb in Germany), as well as Revez, Naltrexona, and Naltrexonum.

The Future of Naltrexone

Researchers continue to explore the potential of naltrexone as a drug and alcohol therapy. Attempts to address compliance issues have resulted in the introduction of a ReVia implant (2003). In addition, Alkermes, Inc. recently developed Vivitrex, a naltrexone injection which lasts a month. (Phase III clinical studies are set to begin in 2005.)

Over the years, researchers have tested naltrexone for a wide variety of medical conditions, including obesity, schizophrenia, and chronic obstructive pulmonary disease. In March 2005, Yale researchers began investigating the use of the Naltrexone to help men and women quit smoking without gaining weight.

The FDA has awarded orphan drug** status to naltrexone to treat symptoms of childhood autism. Another orphan grant has been issued to naltrexone as a therapy for self-injurious behaviors. (Naltrexone therapy for self-injurious behavior is already used extensively in veterinary medicine.)

In addition, researchers have used derivatives of naltrexone to treat other conditions. For example, the FDA granted orphan drug status to methyl-naltrexone as a drug that blocks the side effects of morphine without interfering with pain relief in cancer treatment. (Oncology 1996)

Low Dose Naltrexone

Naltrexone in substantially lower doses (Low Dose Naltrexone) is showing great promise as a treatment for multiple sclerosis, Crohn's disease, AIDS, rheumatoid arthritis, celiac disease, CFIDS, lupus, and certain forms of cancer.

Unfortunately, obtaining FDA approval for LDN will not be a straightforward process. Since naltrexone is now a generic drug, no pharmaceutical company currently holds exclusive manufacturing rights. No company is eager to fund an expensive clinical trial for a drug that will make them so little profit.

However, even without governmental approval or corporate support, LDN is gaining significant grass-roots attention among patients and doctors. The exchange of research information over the internet has greatly accelerated the recognition of the off- label use of LDN.

In the past, the federal government and the pharmaceutical corporations cooperated to create an environment where naltrexone was tested, approved and made available to patients who needed it. Perhaps someday soon they will find a way to do the same for Low Dose Naltrexone .

Last edited 9/16/05
Copyright 2005 by Gazorpa.com

===

*Note on brand names and companies: Naltrexone as used for drug addiction was originally brand-named Trexan. When it was approved for treatment of alcohol dependence, the name was changed to ReVia. In 1991, DuPont and Merck & Co. formed a partnership known as DuPont Merck, which owned the rights to Trexan and ReVia. DuPont Merck marketed ReVia under the name DuPont Pharma. In 2001, Bristol Myers Squibb acquired the rights to ReVia when it acquired DuPont Pharmaceuticals. In 2002, BMS sold the ReVia rights in the US and Canada to Barr Laboratories. Bristol Myers Squibb continues to market ReVia in countries other than the US and Canada.

** Orphan drug status is granted by the FDA to qualifying products intended for the diagnosis, prevention and treatment of rare diseases, or conditions where no current therapy exists, and which affect fewer than 200,000 patients in the US.

Companies developing products that fit this profile may receive help through the Orphan Drug Program in facilitating the development of the product, may be able to gain marketing approval for the product with a smaller amount of data than would usually be required, and may be entitled to seven years of marketing exclusivity upon final FDA marketing approval. Companies may also be eligible to recoup some of the costs of drug development.

To learn more about the orphan drug program, visit the Office of Orphan Products Development at http://www.fda.gov/orphan/.

A major part of the research used to write this article comes from a 2004 case study on developing and marketing medications for drug abuse and addiction published by the US Department of Health and Human Services: http://aspe.hhs. gov/health/reports/cocaine/4cases.htm

From LDNINFO.ORG

Clinical Trials for LDN

Updated: Nov 10, 2008

In Brief

Around the globe, there has been a quantum leap forward in the number of ongoing research studies on LDN. Here is a capsule look at a number of such projects.

Developments that are detailed below:

- A multi-institutional clinical trial of LDN for PPMS in Italy, which includes endorphin measurements, completed in fall 2007, published in September 2008.
- A Phase II placebo-controlled clinical trial of LDN for Crohn's disease at Penn State.
- A Phase II placebo-controlled clinical trial on the efficacy of LDN for children and adolescents with Crohn's disease at Penn State.
- A clinical trial of LDN in HIV-infected citizens of Mali—the first scientific study of LDN for HIV/AIDS in Africa—implemented in October 2007.
- A study of LDN in the treatment of MS at the University of California, San Francisco, implemented in early 2007.
- A clinical trial of LDN in the treatment of fibromyalgia at Stanford Medical Center implemented in October 2007.
- A study by the MindBrain Consortium in Akron, Ohio of, especially, the affective changes in MS treated with LDN, begun late 2007.
- An animal research study at Penn State of naltrexone in a model of a disease that mimics MS, under a small grant from the National MS Society.
- Animal research on neurodegeneration at NIEHS, suggesting a protective role for naltrexone.

Recently Published Clinical Trials of LDN

[Note: use of **boldface**, below, is the website editor's.]

> LDN for MS — Milan, Italy

A long-awaited pilot study of low dose naltrexone therapy in multiple sclerosis was run by the Milan neurological researcher, Dr. Maira Gironi and colleagues. Several northern Italian hospitals began enrolling patients for the study during the first week of December 2006. Dr. Gironi reports that the 6 months of LDN treatment was completed in August 2007. Importantly, Dr. Gironi's research team in Milan has long been a locus for significant research on endorphins in relation to illness, and this study has been tracking accurate assessments of the patients' beta-endorphin levels in response to their LDN treatment.

The subjects were 40 patients affected with Primary Progressive MS. PPMS is an uncommon form of multiple sclerosis that progresses inexorably and for which neurologists have never had an approved treatment to offer.

Results were published in September 2008:

Multiple Sclerosis. 2008 Sep;14(8):1076-83.
A pilot trial of low-dose naltrexone in primary progressive multiple sclerosis.

Gironi M, Martinelli-Boneschi F, Sacerdote P, Solaro C, Zaffaroni M, Cavarretta R, Moiola L, Bucello S, Radaelli M, Pilato V, Rodegher M, Cursi M, Franchi S, Martinelli V, Nemni R, Comi G, Martino G.

Institute of Experimental Neurology (INSPE) and Department of Neurology, San Raffaele Scientific Institute, Via Olgettina 58, Milan, Italy; Fondazione Don Carlo Gnocchi, IRCCS, Milan, Italy.

Abstract: A sixth month phase II multicenter-pilot trial with a low dose of the opiate antagonist Naltrexone (LDN) has been carried out in 40 patients with primary progressive multiple sclerosis (PPMS). The primary end points were safety and tolerability. Secondary outcomes were efficacy on spasticity, pain, fatigue, depression, and quality of life. Clinical and biochemical evaluations were serially performed. Protein concentration of **beta-endorphins (BE)** and mRNA levels and allelic variants of the mu-opiod receptor gene (OPRM1) were analyzed. Five dropouts and two major adverse events occurred. The remaining adverse events did not interfere with daily living. **Neurological disability progressed in only one patient. A significant reduction of spasticity was measured at the end of the trial. BE concentration increased during the trial,** but no association was found between OPRM1 variants and improvement of spasticity. **Our data clearly indicate that LDN is safe and well tolerated in patients with PPMS.**

[Editor's Note: That only one patient showed any progression of PPMS during the six-month period of this trial is extraordinary, as is the occurrence of a statistically significant reduction in spasticity. Two major adverse events were reported but were unassociated with MS or with LDN: one patient had previously unrecognized polycystic kidney disease and the other was diagnosed with metastatic lung cancer.]

Clinical Trials in Progress or Awaiting Publication

> LDN for Crohn's disease—Penn State College of Medicine, Hershey, PA

Dr. Jill Smith's original article, "Low-Dose Naltrexone Therapy Improves Active Crohn's Disease," was published in the Jan 11, 2007 online edition of the American Journal of Gastroenterology (2007;102:1–9) [print edition Apr '07]. This was the first clinical study of LDN published by a US medical journal. Dr. Smith, Professor of Gastroenterology at Pennsylvania State University's College of Medicine, found that two-thirds of the patients in her pilot study went into remission and fully 89% of the group responded to LDN treatment to some degree. She concluded that "LDN therapy appears effective and safe in subjects with active Crohn's disease." That open-label Penn State trial demonstrated the efficacy of LDN in a small group of patients.

As a result, Dr. Smith received an NIH grant that permitted a more definitive Phase II placebo-controlled clinical trial, which by September 2008 had already studied almost all of the 40 patients it plans to include. With just a few patients yet to be added to the study, Dr. Smith is very optimistic about the usefulness of LDN in inflammatory bowel diseases, such as Crohn's disease

Dr. Smith's most recent research on the effects of LDN is a double blind placebo controlled Phase ll study of youngsters from ages 6 to 17 with active Crohn's disease. It was launched at Penn State in July 2008 and is expected to run until July 2010. Participants "will be treated with either naltrexone or placebo for the first 8 weeks then all subjects will receive active naltrexone drug the last 8 weeks." For information about joining the trial, contact Sandra Bingaman, RN, at 717-531-8108 or sbingaman@psu.edu.

> LDN for HIV — Mali, Africa

In September 2007, after years of preparatory efforts by many advocates, the Institutional Review Board in Bamako, the capital of Mali, finally approved plans for a clinical trial of LDN in people who are HIV-infected—the first scientific study of LDN for HIV/AIDS in Africa. Signing up of the volunteer subjects has already begun. The neurologist Dr. Jaquelyn McCandless has taken on the responsibilities of "Expatriate Clinical Monitor" for the medical aspects of the trial.

The study, which is placebo controlled and should last for some 9 months, involves 3 study groups: LDN treatment only; LDN plus antiretroviral drugs; and only antiretroviral drugs. Because of the severe stigma attached to HIV infection in Mali, as of October 2008 the total number of participants who had reached 6 months time in all 3 groups combined amounted only to 16 people. However, Dr. McCandless reported that sign-ups were beginning to improve markedly. The volunteer subjects must be 18 years of age or older and must have reduced CD4 counts in the 350 to 600 cells range at the outset for the LDN treatment only group. The other two groups must begin with CD4 counts below 350 and must be asymptomatic at that time. Laboratory studies are being rechecked at 12-week intervals.

The research team is led by Dr. Abdel Kader Traore and other health officials at the University Hospital in Bamako. Irmat Pharmacy of Manhattan supplied all of the original 4.5mg LDN and matching placebo capsules at no cost. However, due to untranslated English-French communications, the study was approved for 3mg LDN dosage, and that is being supplied by Skip's Pharmacy of Boca Raton. In addition, the plans include careful attention to counseling aimed at improving preventive health practices for women and children. Both Dr. McCandless and her colleague husband, Jack Zimmerman, plan to be in Mali from time to time to supervise the study.

Dr. McCandless is actively seeking philanthropic donations - jmccandless@prodigy.net

The Fourth LDN Conference of October 2008 was proud to be able to donate $5,595 dollars from voluntary individual contributions.

> LDN for MS—University of California, San Francisco, CA

A study of LDN in the treatment of MS at the University of California, San Francisco, was implemented in early 2007 by neurological researcher Bruce Cree, MD, and colleagues. Some 80 patients with MS were involved in this double-blind, "Randomized, Placebo-Controlled, Crossover-Design Study of the Effects of Low Dose Naltrexone on Quality of Life as Measured by the Multiple Sclerosis Quality of Life Inventory." Each subject received either LDN or a placebo for 8 weeks, followed by one week without either, and then a further 8 weeks on the the alternate capsule. A substantial contribution toward the study has been made by the the the LDN for MS Research Fund.

Dr. Cree reported the conclusions as follows in a poster presentation to the World Congress on Treatment and Research in Multiple Sclerosis, held in September 2008 in Montreal, Canada. His report still awaited publication at that date:

Conclusions

- 8 weeks of treatment with LDN significantly improved quality of life indices for mental health, pain, and self-reported cognitive function of MS patients as measured by the MSQLI [MS Quality of Life Inventory]
- An impact on physical quality of life indices including fatigue, bowel and bladder control, sexual satisfaction, and visual function was not observed
- The benefits of LDN were not affected by disease course, age, treatment order, or treatment with either interferon beta or Copaxone
- The only treatment related adverse event reported was vivid dreaming during the first week of the study drug in some patients
- Potential effects of LDN beyond 8 weeks of treatment were not addressed in this study
- Multicenter randomized clinical trials of LDN in MS are warranted

Dr. Cree also included the following in his Acknowledgment:

We are grateful to the MS patients for participating in this study and wish to specially acknowledge the efforts of SammyJo Wilkinson of ldners.org and the other fundraisers who made this trial possible. To our knowledge, this is the first patient-funded clinical trial in MS.

> LDN for Fibromyalgia — Stanford, California

A single-blind, small clinical trial of LDN for the treatment of fibromyalgia was begun at Stanford Medical Center in June 2007; principal Investigator Sean Mackey and sub-investigator Jarred Younger. In September 2008, Younger advised us as follows:

The LDN trial on 10 individuals gave us encouraging results, which we hope to publish in the next 2-3 months. The findings warrant a larger, double-blind trial, planning for which is currently ongoing. We are actively recruiting individuals with fibromyalgia in the San Francisco Bay area to participate in the second study. **We are also pursuing a small trial of LDN for pediatric fibromyalgia patients.** While I can't talk about specific results, I will say that the majority of our study participants asked to continue taking LDN after the conclusion of the study. Side-effects were virtually non-existent, with 2 reports of increased vividness of dreams, and 1 report of transient insomnia.

Additional information can be found at:
http://www.clinicaltrials.gov/ct2/show/NCT00568555?term=fibromyalgia&rank=63.

> LDN for MS — Akron, Ohio

In May 2007, the MindBrain Consortium and the Department of Psychiatry of Summa Hospital System of Akron, Ohio, along with the nearby Oak Clinic for the treatment of Multiple Sclerosis, announced a new scientific study of the effects of treating MS with low dose naltrexone. Psychologist David Pincus and his colleagues coordinated the study. It was a 16 week, double-blind, randomized, placebo-controlled, crossover-design analysis of 36 patients with either progressive or relapsing-remitting MS. The study examined symptom severity as well as any changes in quality of life, sleep patterns, and affective states.

In early October 2007, Dr. Pincus wrote as follows:

We have enrolled more than 20 of the 36 people intended; we expect to be fully recruited within the next 3 or 4 weeks, and, three months following the end of enrollment we will have all the data. The study is going well, a couple of people have dropped out or been removed for one reason or another, but none because of a problem with sleep. One patient had sleeping issues for a few nights, but then has been ok. We are looking at the psychoactive properties of LDN as well as assessing improvement of MS symptoms, and hope to find some changes in perception of energy level that correlate with personality type and amount of dreaming reported.

One year later, Dr. Pincus reported problematic outcomes in his study, with little apparent differences between the placebo and treatment groups. After lengthy consideration with his colleagues, he wrote as follows:

We did not exclude patients on existing immunosuppressants....The existing immunosuppressants may have inhibited the LDN effects in this population.

Animal Trials of LDN

> Research on Neurodegeneration at NIEHS Suggests a Protective Naltrexone Role

J.S. Hong, Ph.D., head of the Neuropharmacology Section of the Laboratory of Pharmacology and Chemistry at the National Institute of Environmental Health Sciences, finds that "morphinan" drugs, including naltrexone and naloxone, are able to reduce inflammatory reactions in microglia brain cells in animal studies. Such inflammation is believed to be central to the progressive neurodegenerative effects seen in disorders such as Parkinson's disease and Alzheimer's disease. Hong's report, summarizing the role of microglia in inflammation-related neurodegeneration and the potential of therapy using morphinans, appears in a January 2007 issue of *Nature Reviews Neuroscience* [8(1):57-69].

> Research at Penn State: LDN for an Animal Model of MS

The National Multiple Sclerosis Society "awarded a small Pilot Award to Ian Zagon [Ph.D.] at Pennsylvania State University in Hershey, PA for the term of 09/01/2006 through 08/31/2007 in the amount of $44,000. The title of his project is 'Role of opioid peptides and receptors in MS.' This study [treated] an animal model of MS daily with either a high dose of naltrexone or a low dose of naltrexone to determine whether naltrexone influences disease course."

Zagon described the project as follows:

This research project raises the question of whether endogenous opioids and opioid receptors influence the course of MS. This is a novel and innovative concept that is valuable to explore. To test this hypothesis, we will subject [rodents] to experimental autoimmune encephalomyelitis (EAE), a model that mimics MS. Animals will be treated daily with a high dose of [naltrexone] (HDN) or a low dose of [naltrexone] (LDN)....Our expectations are that continuous opioid receptor blockade will exacerbate the progression of MS, whereas a low dose of naltrexone will retard the course of this disease. Evidence for the involvement of endogenous opioids and opioid receptors in

MS will open a new field of research related to the pathogenesis of this disease, and contribute to the development of strategies for treatment.

Dr. Zagon's expectations were met, as is clear in the titles of the two poster presentations (below), which he gave to the World Congress on Treatment and Research in Multiple Sclerosis, held in September 2008 in Montreal, Canada. The actual data still awaited journal publication at that date:

Poster 190—**Low-dose naltrexone (LDN) prevents development or delays onset and reduces severity of experimental autoimmune encephalomyelitis in mice.** K. Rahn, P. McLaughlin (Hershey, Pennsylvania, USA), R. Bonneau, A. Turel, G. Thomas, I. Zagon.

Poster 216—**The complete blockade of opioid receptors with naltrexone exacerbates experimental autoimmune encephalomyelitis in a mouse model.** I. Zagon (Hershey, Pennsylvania, USA), K. Rahn, R. Bonneau, A. Turel, G. Thomas, P. McLaughlin.

Past Completed Clinical Trials of Low Dose Naltrexone

> Penn State Trial for Crohn's Disease

Endoscopic Improvement in Crohn's Colitis with Naltrexone

The report on this groundbreaking research—**"Low-Dose Naltrexone as a Treatment For Active Crohn's Disease"**—was presented on May 23, 2006 at Digestive Diseases Week, a prestigious gastrointestinal conference, by Professor Jill Smith of the Pennsylvania State University College of Medicine. Dr. Smith's research paper, "Low-Dose Naltrexone Therapy Improves Active Crohn's Disease," has been published by the *American Journal of Gastroenterology* in its January 11, 2007 edition.

Dr. Smith and her colleagues concluded that "LDN therapy offers an alternative safe, effective, and economic means of treating subjects with active Crohn's disease."

According to the news from Penn State, the National Institutes of Health has already granted $500,000 for Dr. Smith's group to continue the study. This funding should help assure a full-fledged placebo-controlled scientific trial of LDN in Crohn's disease. (Notably, Dr. Smith and her research teams are also involved in exploring the direct effects of using a form of endorphin by infusion in order to treat pancreatic and colon cancer.)

Below are some extracts from the trial summary that was published online by the gastroenterology conference:

Low-Dose Naltrexone as a Treatment For Active Crohn's Disease

J. P. Smith[1]; H. E. Stock[1]; S. I. Bingaman[1]; D. T. Mauger[2]; I. S. Zagon[3]

1. Medicine, The Pennsylvania State University College of Medicine, Hershey, PA, USA.
2. Health Evaluation Sciences, The Pennsylvania State University College of Medicine, Hershey, PA, USA.
3. Neural and Behavioral Sciences, The Pennsylvania State University College of Medicine, Hershey, PA, USA.

Methods: Eligible subjects with histologically and endoscopically confirmed active Crohn's disease with a Crohn's Activity Index (CDAI) score of 220-450 were enrolled in a study using 4.5 mg naltrexone/day. Subjects were required to be off infliximab for at least 8-weeks, and this medication was not allowed during the trial. Other drug therapy for Crohn's disease utilized 4 or more weeks prior to enrollment was continued at the same dosages.... Drug [LDN] was administered orally each evening for a 12-week period. Laboratory tests, erythrocyte sedimentation rates, C-Reactive protein, and CDAI scores were assessed monthly and 4 weeks after discontinuing the medication.

Results: Seventeen patients with a mean initial CDAI[*] score of 356 ± 27 were enrolled in the study. CDAI scores decreased significantly ($p<0.01$) with LDN, and remained statistically lower than baseline 4-weeks after completing therapy (see Figure).

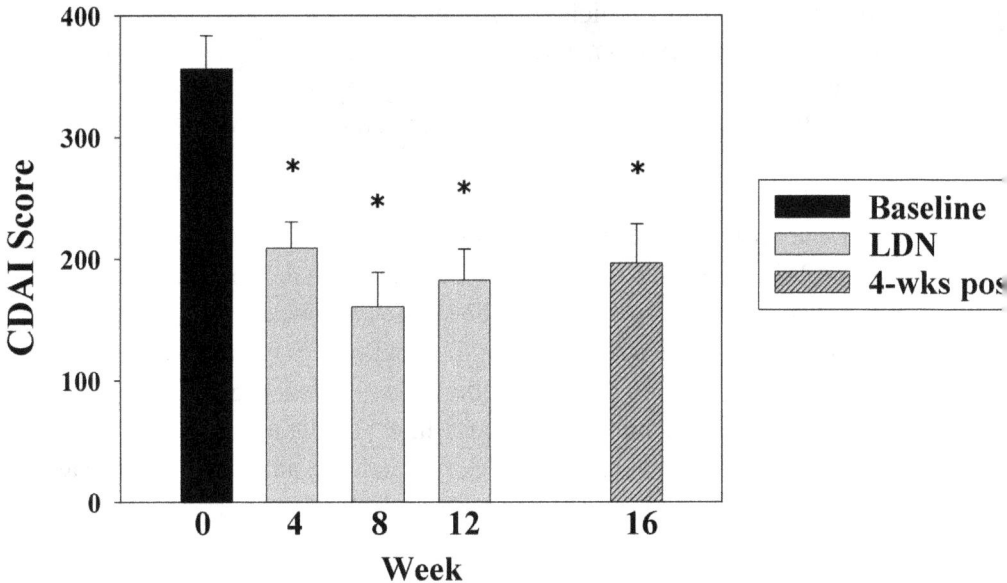

Eighty-nine percent of patients exhibited a response to therapy (>70-point decrease in CDAI, p<0.001) and 67% achieved remission (CDAI score <150). QOL* surveys indicated marked improvement with LDN. No laboratory abnormalities were noted. One subject undergoing routine endoscopic procedures showed healing of the intestinal mucosa. In both subjects with open fistulas, closure was noted with LDN. The most common side effect of LDN was sleep disturbances (7 patients).

Conclusions: **LDN therapy offers an alternative safe, effective, and economic means of treating subjects with active Crohn's disease.**

QOL = Quality of Life] [Editor's Note: CDAI = Crohn's Disease Activity Index;

> Pain Therapeutics Ends Irritable Bowel Syndrome Trials of Ultra-low Naltrexone Dosage

In December 2005, Pain Therapeutics, Inc. announced results of its Phase III study with PTI-901. [Editor's Note: PTI-901 contains only

0.5mg of naltrexone, which is well below the therapeutic dosage range for LDN—normally from 1.75mg to 4.5mg every night. LDN in the normal dosage range has been anecdotally reported quite beneficial in halting IBS.] Excerpt from PTI's announcement:

This randomized, double-blinded, multi-center U.S. study compared a daily dose of PTI-901 against placebo in 600 women with documented IBS over a three-month treatment period. PTI-901 showed a favorable safety profile and patients reported statistically meaningful relief of IBS symptoms in the second month of treatment (p<0.02), but the drug did not demonstrate a meaningful benefit in the third month of treatment, which was defined as the primary endpoint. According to current regulatory standards, an experimental drug for chronic IBS needs to show efficacy at the end of a three-month treatment period.

The Company believes this study was well designed to detect any durable benefits of PTI-901 versus placebo in a large patient population with IBS. Based on the adequacy of the study itself, coupled with today's clinical results, the Company is discontinuing all further clinical development activities with PTI-901.

> Dr. Evers Trial in Germany for Multiple Sclerosis (MS)

Conducted in the Multiple Sclerosis Clinic of Dr. Evers Hospital in Sundern, Germany, the starting date was October 15, 2004. It is described as a short-term scientific, randomized, placebo-controlled, double-blind study involving patients with either secondary-progressive MS (SPMS) or primary-progressive MS (PPMS).

[Editor's Note: Unfortunately, because of some early complaints of sleep disturbance, the principal investigator of this trial switched all of the study group to taking LDN at 9am in the morning, a questionable dosage time. It is generally recognized that the most effective time to take LDN is at bedtime, between 9pm and 3am, due to the fact that the endorphins for each day are always produced at their peak rate in the pre-dawn hours. A 9am dosage time, as was used in this trial, might conceivably suppress—rather than boost—a patient's immune system.]

The purpose of the study was to investigate what MS-associated symptoms are positively influenced by LDN (low dose naltrexone, 3 mg per day). The principal investigator, Dr. Mir, reported his findings at the First Annual LDN Conference in 2005, as well as on his website, http://www.klinik-dr-evers.de/.

www.ingramcontent.com/pod-product-compliance
Lightning Source LLC
Chambersburg PA
CBHW070805270326
41927CB00010B/2296